Human Existence, Medicine and Ethics

Reflections on Human Life

Human Existence, Medicine and Ethics

Reflections on Human Life

William E. May
Associate Professor of Moral Theology
The Catholic University of America
Washington, D.C.

FRANCISCAN HERALD PRESS

1434 West 51st Street   Chicago, Illinois 60609

Library of Congress Cataloging in Publication Data

May, William E.   1928-
  Human existence, medicine, and ethics.

  Includes bibliographical references and index.
  1. Medical ethics. 2. Christian ethics—Catholic
authors. I. Title. [DNLM: 1. Catholicism.
2. Ethics, Medical. W50 M466h]
R724.M28   174′.2   77-8149
ISBN 0-8199-0677-8

NIHIL OBSTAT:
Mark Hegener O.F.M.
Censor Deputatus

IMPRIMATUR:
✠William Cardinal Baum
Archbishop of Washington, D.C.

September 8, 1977
Feast of the Nativity of the Blessed Virgin Mary

MADE IN THE UNITED STATES OF AMERICA

To my children, Michael, Mary Patricia, Thomas,
Timothy, Patrick, Susan, and Kathleen, and to all
in their generation

Acknowledgments

This book offers reflections on the meaning of human life, in its beginning, its care, and its end, in light of contemporary developments in the biomedical sciences. Although many important questions are not considered, for example, organ transplants from living donors and the allocation of sparse medical resources, those that are considered deeply touch the meaning of human existence.

I am indebted to many persons for the help they gave me in finishing this work: my students, both undergraduate and graduate, at The Catholic University of America; Dr. Warren T. Reich of the Center for Bioethics of the Kennedy Institute at Georgetown University and Sister Jean W. Hitzeman O.P., a doctor in biology and director of studies for the Adrian Dominicans, who read early drafts and offered kindly corrections and suggestions; the Reverend Donald McCarthy of Mt. St. Mary's Seminary of the West, Norwood, Ohio, who read the manuscript from which this text emerged and made many constructive suggestions; the Reverend Mark Hegener O.F.M. of the Franciscan Herald Press, who gave me encouragement and advice; and above all my wife, Patricia, a mother, nurse, and Montessori educator, who shares my deep interest in the topics of this book and gives me an example of one who loves life and cares for persons. I am grateful also to my colleagues in moral philosophy and Christian ethics, in particular Germain Grisez and Paul Ramsey, whose work and thought have been of tremendous influence on me.

Finally, I thank the editors of *Linacre Quarterly* for allowing me to adapt, in chapter 1, material that originally appeared in that quarterly.

Contents

Introduction: Christian Faith, Human Existence, and Human Acts

The following chapters attempt to understand the moral questions raised by some biomedical technologies that are now available or soon will be. They are concerned with human activities and practices that pertain to the generation, care, and termination of human existence and their impact upon persons and societies.

This Introduction is concerned with the human beings who are or will be either the agents of these acts of generating, caring for, and terminating human existence or the subjects who are or will be affected by them.

The basic reason why we are interested in these questions is that we are interested in ourselves. We want to know who we are and what we are to do if we are to be the kind of beings we are meant to be.[1]

Here I want to offer some reflections, rooted in Christian faith, on the meaning of human existence and the significance of human acts. My purpose is to articulate an understanding of human existence and human acts that is grounded in Christian faith and taught by the Church, so that readers will be able to understand the perspective within which the questions will be addressed.

Christian Understanding of God and of Human Beings

The way a Christian understands God and human existence can perhaps be initially appreciated by contrasting the thought

1

of Aristotle, the great Greek philosopher, with the faith of the Christian. For Aristotle, man's highest good, the *summum bonum*, is happiness, and this is a good that all men by nature desire.[2] This is also a good "achievable by action" and immanent in human life here and now,[3] consisting principally in wisdom, virtue, and pleasure. For him the perfect and happy life, achieved by virtuous activity, is "the most blessed and beautiful of things, and also that which gives the greatest joy."[4] Moreover, he considered friendship between man and God to be impossible, an utterly absurd and foolish notion. "It would be ridiculous," Aristotle wrote, "to reproach God because the love we receive from him in return is not equal to the love we give him, just as it would be ridiculous for the subject to make a similar reproach to his prince. For it is the role of the prince to receive love, not to give it."[5]

For the Christian, on the other hand, God alone is the highest good, the *summum bonum*. For the Christian the one and only God, the living God of history, is "wholly other" than man and all creation. He is utterly transcendent and is the good that must be loved above all other goods. But for the Christian this supremely transcendent being is first and foremost, as Karl Barth has noted so eloquently, a God who

> exists neither *next* to man nor merely *above* him, but rather *with* him, *by* him, and most important of all, *for* him. He is man's God not only as Lord but also as father, brother, friend; and this relationship implies neither a diminution nor in any way a denial, but instead, a confirmation of his divine essence itself.[6]

In the Christian tradition the utterly supreme good, God, is a personal being who has made man for himself. To be a human being means, in this tradition, to be a being with a vocation and a destiny, life in communion with the *summum bonum*, a life that he *wills* to share with us, his children.[7] In this tradition, to be a human being is to be a child of God, to be called to exist in a union of friendship with God himself. We are human beings, of whom it is written: "Does a woman forget her baby at the breast, or fail to cherish the son of her womb? Yet even if they forget, I will never forget you. See, I have branded you on the palms of my hands" (Is 49:15–16). Augustine well expressed this Christian view of human existence: "You have made us for yourself, O Lord, and our hearts are restless until they rest in you."[8]

The love that God has for his children was supremely revealed in the life, death, and resurrection of Jesus, in whom he became one with us so that we could become one with him.[9] Jesus, the Uncreated Word of the Father becomes man, becomes one of us to live with us and for us, is both the definitive revelation of the Father, the epiphany of God, and the one who tells us who we are. He tells us that the one and only God, the good whom we are to love above all other goods, is the best friend we can ever have, the one who will never betray us no matter how terribly we may betray him. Because of Jesus we can make Paul's words our own: "For I am certain of this: neither death nor life, no angel, no prince, nothing that exists, nothing still to come, not any power, or height or depth, nor any created thing, can ever come between us and the love of God made visible in Christ Jesus our Lord" (Rom 8:38–39). God, manifested in and through Jesus, is, in other words, true to his word. So true to his word is God that, through his word, he has given us himself irrevocably, for his definitive word to us is his Uncreated Word, the word who "made his dwelling among us . . . filled with enduring love" (Jn 1:14), the word who "became flesh," who came to share our humanity so that he might enable us to share his divinity.[10]

The God of Christian faith is, moreover, absolutely innocent of evil.[11] He wills for us only the good; in fact, he wills for us *the* good, himself, for he has made us to be the kind of beings with whom he can share his life and he has made it possible for us, through his love, to participate in that life. Evil exists, and this sovereignly perfect being and loving friend permits it to be, but he does so only that from it he may draw an even greater good.[12]

Jesus, Christians believe, not only tells us who God is, he also tells us who *we* are. Not only are we beings made in the image of God (Gn 1:27), that is, living images or icons of God, we are also God's children: "What love the Father has bestowed on us by letting us be called children of God! Yet that is what we are"

(1 Jn 3:1). Indeed, because God himself has become one of us in and through Jesus, the Christian believes that to be a human being is to be precisely that kind of being that "God himself becomes (though remaining God) when he exteriorizes himself into the dimension of what is other than himself, the non-divine."[13]

This is the great truth about human existence that is mediated through Christian faith. It can perhaps be expressed this way: to be a human being is to be a word uttered by the living and loving God. We are the created words that God's Uncreated Word became. Each human being is a living word, spoken by God himself and addressed by him to other human beings. Each human being, moreover, precisely because he or she is a living word spoken by God, is irreplaceable, precious, priceless. To be a human being, accordingly, is to be a *being of moral worth*. This means that every human being is the subject of inalienable rights that are to be recognized by others and that demand legal protection by society. It means that every human being has a dignity that is a created participation in the infinite dignity, indeed sanctity, of God himself.[14] It means that every human being, precisely in virtue of being a human being, transcends or surpasses the society in which he or she lives and, as a consequence, can never rightly be considered simply a part related to some larger whole. It means, in other words, that membership in the human species is of transcendent moral significance.

Corporate or Covenantal Character of Human Existence

The Christian believes, in addition, that a human being is meant to exist within a human community. The life that God wills to share with each of us personally is not given to us simply as individuals, as isolated entities. Rather, it is personally extended to each of us as members of a people, of a community ultimately reaching out to include all human beings, with whom God has allied or "covenanted" himself, a people whom he has made his own because of his surpassing love.[15] In biblical and Christian faith, a human being is never understood simply as an individual but as one who is meant to exist *with* and *needs* to exist with other human beings if he or she is to grow to realize the potential that he or she has by virtue of being a human being.

Vatican II expressed this belief as follows: "The progress of the human person and the advance of society itself hinge on each other . . . social life is not something added on to man. Through his dealing with others, through reciprocal duties, and through fraternal dialogue he develops all his gifts and is able to rise to his destiny."[16]

By reason of being the living words of God, we are beings of moral worth. But we come to know who we are and we develop the capabilities we possess because we are his living words only in company with our fellow words, our fellow human beings. Our lives as God's words are inextricably linked to the lives of others and our personal identity is bound up with the identities of the various communities in which we live and move and have our being, for we discover ourselves, we find out who we are and what we are to do, in our relationships with others.

The corporate—or better, covenantal—character of our existence as living words needs to be probed more deeply. None of us—no human being anywhere—was a *moral being* at conception or even at birth. But each of us was a *being of moral worth* from the very beginning of his existence and was radically capable, precisely because he was a being of moral worth or a living word of God, of becoming a moral being, that is, a being capable of coming to know his identity and freely shaping his life by acting in response to his knowledge of what it means to be a human being. A moral being is one who is able to tell right from wrong, to distinguish *is* from *ought,* and capable of self-determination. A moral being bears duties and obligations as well as rights and dignity. All human beings, the Christian believes, are of moral worth, bearers of inalienable rights. Ultimately, most human beings *become* moral beings, bearers of obligations, because being living words of God capacitates them for acting intelligently and freely, but they actually become moral beings or moral agents because others have given them the opportunity to develop these capacities.

Some human beings never become moral beings, either because

they die in infancy or childhood, before they can develop their ability to think and freely choose for themselves the life they are to lead, or because of some pathological condition. Still others, who were once moral beings, cease to be so because of illness or old age. But all of them, the Christian believes, are and remain beings of moral worth, precious in the sight of the Lord, for whom Jesus gave his life and to whom he wills to bring the glory of the resurrection.

All of this helps show us the meaning of our existence as a covenantal existence. If a human being, a living word of God himself, is to develop the capacities he has by virtue of being what he is, he needs help, he needs a friend, he needs love. We know that God is ready to give us his help and friendship, but he wills to give it to us through our fellow words, our fellow human beings. The life he wills to share with us is a gift, given personally to each of us by God himself, but he wills to mediate this gift of life and love through a human community.

No one, including the writer, would have any notion of himself as a moral being, or even as a self, had it not been for the help of others. No one lifts himself to the level of moral existence by his own bootstraps, as it were. Rather, we achieve such elevation with the help of the human community, the community of our fellow words, which, first of all, *lets us be* and then *enables* us to be ourselves. Thus our existence as human beings is meant to be not only a being *with* others, a coexistence, but, more importantly, a being *for* others, a "for-existence." God, the Christian believes, is the being who is both with and for us. We, his living icons and created words, are therefore meant to be beings who exist both with and for our fellow words.[17]

Sin and the Covenant

The meaning of human existence as that of a being with and for our fellow words is strikingly illustrated in the Christian tradition by the teaching on sin. In its essence, sin is an ineradicable expression of the whole person; it wells up from one's "heart," from the inner core of one's existence. Not only does "a good man draw what is good from the store of goodness in his heart" (Lk 6:45), it is, Jesus teaches us, "what comes out of a man that makes him unclean. For it is from within, from man's heart, that evil intentions emerge; fornication, theft, murder, adultery, avarice, malice, deceit, indecency, envy, slander, pride, folly. All these evil things come from within and make a man unclean" (Mk 7:21–23).

At root, sin is an unwillingness to submit to God; as such, it is an expression of human freedom, of our capacity to give to ourselves, through our choices, an attitude and a definitive being.[18] As an act expressive of our personality, sin is a nay-saying to God; it is a refusal to accept his gift of himself, a rejection of the life that he wills to share with us.[19]

Sin ultimately is self-destruction that we bring upon ourselves by our free choices. But sin is not purely negative, it is not a nothing; there is something positive in every sin. Like all evil, sin is a deprivation of the being that *ought* to be present. From the very beginning, the sinful deed we choose is more than a striving for self-destruction. The person who sins performs "an essentially ambivalent action. He strives toward some good and he tries to realize a value, but he does so against God's covenant and order, thus operating in a negative, destructive way . . . sin is negative, but it renders its denial concrete in a positive action. Even the most direct hardening against God and one's fellow man remains a self-affirmation, a positing of one's own freedom."[20]

Sin expresses our personal rejection of God and the life—his very own life—that he wills to communicate to us; it is also a rupturing of the covenantal relationship between God and man and among men: it also destroys the friendship that he wants to give us and that he wants to exist in and among men. Because we are not simply individuals but persons, that is, personal subjects existing within a community of fellow subjects, every sin has social results. Our personal sins affect not only us but other human beings and the fabric of our lives together. As a result of sin we are alienated from or made strangers not only to God but to our fellow words as well, and even to ourselves.[21] As a result of personal sins—none of us is without sin, for "if we say we have no sin in us, we are deceiving ourselves and refusing to admit the truth" (1 Jn 1:8)—the world is wounded by sin, broken by sin. We find ourselves unable to love and at a loss to understand ourselves, and unable, as Paul tells us, "to carry out the things I want to do" but, instead, doing the very things we hate (Rom 7:15). Sin cripples us in our struggle to know who we are and what we are to do, and then in our endeavor to do what we know we are to do.

We can summarize the understanding of God and of human existence, mediated by Christian faith, in the following way. God, the *summum bonum,* the good that is to be loved above all other goods, made us to share his very own life. Because he made us for this purpose, we are in truth his images; we are his created words, and his Uncreated Word became, like us, a created word, a human being. Because we are his living images we are beings of moral worth; and because we are radically capable, by virtue of being his images and words, of becoming conscious of ourselves and of the meaning of our actions, we are capable of becoming moral beings, moral agents. We are radically capable of determining our own lives and establishing our own identity through our own choices.

We make these choices after a process of deliberation in which we struggle to come to a true understanding of ourselves and our lives; and, because of our freedom, we can choose to act in a way that contradicts our true understanding of who we are and what we are to do if we are to be living and faithful images of God. Our freedom allows us to reject God's offer of life by refusing to be his faithful images, by hardening our hearts against him and our fellow words.

So greatly does God love us, however, that he has become one with us in Jesus, the man born of woman, whom we confess to be our Lord and Redeemer, the man who is indeed God's definitive word to us and reveals that we can be ourselves only if we are willing, like him, to be not only *with* our fellow words but *for* them as well—that we can be true words of the Father only if we are willing, as his Uncreated Word was willing, to be the servants of our fellow words and unwilling to choose to do any deed that is targeted on destroying a good in them to which they have a claim, a right, as beings of moral worth.

Significance of Human Acts

The vocation and destiny of every human being is life with God, the *summum bonum,* who is to be loved above every other good. God freely wills to give us a life of loving friendship, but he cannot give his life and love to us unless we freely choose to receive his gift. He made us to be the kind of beings we are, his living words, precisely so there could be beings with whom he could share his life and love.[22] But he cannot force his friendship on us; the very notion is absurd. Just as I cannot order my wife to accept my love, compel her to receive it, neither can God order or compel us to receive his gift of himself. It is a gift freely given, and for it to remain a gift it must be freely received. We must, if we are to love God, freely choose to do so.

But how do we freely accept God's gift of love and give him our love in return? We do so by our willingness to do what we come to know we must do if we are to be his faithful images, his loving words, and by our unwillingness to do what we come to know we ought not do if we are to be true to him. In other words, we determine our lives and give ourselves a definitive moral identity by the kinds of deeds we freely choose to do.

This means that a Christian is interested in human acts, human deeds, not so much because of what they "get done" but because of what they "get said."[23] We are interested in human acts insofar as they have something to say about ourselves, insofar as they manifest our identity and insofar as we make ourselves what we become in and through the deeds we choose to do.

It is for this reason that the Church, since the days of St. Paul (cf. Rom 3:8),[24] has consistently opposed the view that the end justifies the means. By this the Church means that a good end, for example, the well-being and happiness of many, can never justify a means, an act, that is itself evil because reality- or truth-making factors are discernible within the deed that make it evil.

The point I am trying to make can be clarified if we reflect for a moment on human identity. A human being, through his free choices, can give himself a definite identity as a moral being. The Christian believes that a human being, who is the living image and word of God, ought not to take on himself the identity of an evildoer, for instance, the identity of a killer or liar or adulterer or exploiter of the weak. But how does a human being become a killer, an adulterer, a liar, an exploiter? By being willing to choose to do acts that are truly acts of killing, adultery, lying, exploiting.

Thus the Christian is enormously interested in the significance or meaning or intelligibility of human acts.[25] But to describe human acts truthfully is no easy task. The Christian has the teaching of the Church to guide him, but it is the personal responsibility of each Christian—indeed, of every human being who has become a moral agent—to seek conscientiously to get to a true understanding of his acts.

A full discussion of this very important subject[26] is not possible here, but we can outline a basic approach for understanding the significance of human acts. This approach is rooted in the Christian tradition, particularly in the thought of St. Thomas Aquinas, and is reflected in the writings of some contemporary moral theologians and philosophers. Its basic features have been most adequately developed in the contemporary world, in my judgment, by Germain Grisez,[27] and in the remainder of this Introduction I will simply endeavor to delineate its general character and show why I believe it is in accord with a Christian understanding of human existence and the meaning of human acts.

According to this approach there are certain basic human goods, such as life and health, truth, friendship, justice, and peace. Each of these goods is a real good of human persons, rooted in real needs of human persons. Each of these goods, which together are constitutive of what can be termed the *totum bonum humanum,*[28] is a good to be *prized,* not *priced;* each is a good *of* human beings, not *for* human beings; each is a good in itself, not a merely useful good; each is a human personal good, corresponding to a dimension of our being as beings of moral worth.[29] Each is a created participation of the goodness of God himself, the *summum bonum.*

We come to know these goods through experience and through reflecting upon experience.[30] As consciously apprehended, each of these goods functions as a principle of intelligent behavior, or what Aquinas termed a first principle of practical reason,[31] inasmuch as each of these goods orients us toward something that is authentically worthy of choice, something that "is to be" through our deeds, a good that is not only achievable by action but a good in which we participate, in and through our actions.

Because each of these goods is a basic human good, something that is really good if we are to be fully the kind of beings we are meant to be, we ought to respect them for what they are. We ought to love these goods and be willing to affirm them both in ourselves and in our fellow words of God, recognizing in them the realities that bring us the fullness of being, realities that correspond to needs that exist in us simply because we are human beings.[32]

If this is so, we ought not, of set purpose, seek to destroy these goods, either in ourselves or in others. We ought not, in other words, consider them as being no longer good here and now, as no longer worthy of our love and respect. In short, we ought not, in and through our actions, set our wills, our person, against these goods of set purpose and, of direct intent, seek their destruction.[33]

None of these basic human goods is the *summum bonum,* the be-all and end-all of life, an absolute good in this sense. God alone is the *summum bonum.* But each of these basic human goods is a good, that is, something worthy of human choice and a created participation in the goodness of that uncreated good, God, who *is* the *summum bonum.* When we are enjoined by the biblical writers and by Jesus to be of clean heart, this means that we are to be open to these goods of human beings and to their realization both in ourselves and others. It means that we are to be ready to recognize these goods for what they are, real goods of human beings, and to be unwilling to set out, in and through our deeds, precisely to destroy these goods in human beings.

Thus, in this view, a human being cannot rightfully choose to do a deed that is destructive in and of itself, and in such a way that it cannot *not* be intended to be destructive, of a basic human good such as life. At times a human being may choose to do a deed in which a basic human good, such as life, is destroyed, but one can rightfully choose to do this only when both the agent's intent and the thrust of the act are targeted on a good achievable in and through the deed. In such instances the evil caused is an inevitable, unavoidable, and partial aspect of the entire human act, and the evil is an aspect that is *not* intended by the doer but is permitted by him because of some proportionately serious reason.[34] Such deeds may be directly destructive of a human good in the order of physical causality, but they are not directly destructive of a human good in the order of human activity and intentionality inasmuch as they are neither intended directly (but only foreseen and permitted) nor targeted on the achievement of the evil.

This approach to describing human acts truthfully, to getting at their intelligibility, seriously evaluates the meaning of our acts as revelatory of our moral identity. It holds that as a human being, as an image of God and word of God, I ought *not* be willing to choose to do a deed that will require, as an inevitable necessity, that I be willing to set myself in my will (biblically, my "heart") against a real good of another human being, another being of moral worth—that requires me to say of these goods, here and now, that they are nongoods, no longer worthy of my love. For the goods in question (life, health, justice, peace, friendship, and whatever else comprise the whole human good) are not abstractions but realities that together make up the total good of human beings and are rooted in the *being* of those precious and priceless beings with whom and for whom we are to live, namely, our fellow images and words of God.

This approach will be illustrated when we take up specific questions. The chief point here is that, in a Christian understanding of human existence, the intelligibility or meaning of human deeds is of paramount significance. For it is in and through the deeds that we freely choose to do what we respond to God's summons to choose life, to accept his gift of friendship. We "make or break" our lives by the deeds we choose to do, and we know their significance not by looking at their results but at the deeds themselves and what they tell us about ourselves.

Introduction

1. This is a point perceptively made by Walter Mondale in a speech on the Senate floor (before he became Vice President), urging the establishment of a National Advisory Commission on Health, Science, and Society. The senator declared: "There is another matter

perhaps more profound [than the vexing problems of a practical nature raised by scientific advances]. The biomedical technologies work directly on man's biological nature, including those aspects long regarded as most distinctively human. Thus we should expect major challenges to our traditional image of man as this technology unfolds. The impact upon our ideas of free will, birth and death, and the good life is likely to be even more staggering than any actual manipulations performed with the new technologies." Reprinted in *Hastings Center Report,* 1 (June 1971): 1–2.

2. Aristotle, *Nicomachean Ethics,* I, 7, 1097a 33–1097b 11.

3. On the good achievable by action see *ibid.,* I, 7, 1097b 22–24; on the immanence of happiness in human life here and now see *ibid.,* X, 7, 1177a 12–28.

4. *Eudemean Ethics,* I, 1, 1214a 8–9.

5. *Ibid.,* VII, 3, 1238b 26–29.

6. Karl Barth, *Evangelical Theology: An Introduction* (New York: Holt, Rinehart and Winston, 1963), p. 11.

7. On this see the teaching of Vatican II in *Gaudium et Spes* [Pastoral Constitution on the Church Today], pars. 15–17.

8. St. Augustine, *Confessions,* I, 1.

9. See *Gaudium et Spes,* par. 22.

10. This is a truth daily brought to mind in the Mass, when, during the preparation of our gifts, water is mixed with wine as we pray: "By the mystery of this water and wine may we come to share in the divinity of Christ, who humbled himself to share in our humanity."

11. On this see *Gaudium et Spes,* par. 19. See also the penetrating study by Jacques Maritain, *God and the Permission of Evil* (Milwaukee: Bruce, 1967).

12. See *Gaudium et Spes,* pars. 19–22.

13. Karl Rahner, "On the Theology of the Incarnation," in *Theological Investigations* (Baltimore: Helicon, 1966), Vol. 4, p. 107.

14. On this see *Gaudium et Spes,* par. 75.

15. On the central notion of covenant in biblical and Christian thought see Jean Giblet and Pierre Grelot, "Covenant," in *Dictionary of Biblical Theology,* ed. Xavier Leon-Dufour (New York: Desclée, 1967), pp. 75–79.

16. *Gaudium et Spes,* par. 25.

17. On this see Rahner, *loc. cit.,* pp. 111–116.

18. On this see Piet Schoonenberg, *Man and Sin* (Notre Dame, Ind.: University of Notre Dame Press, 1965), pp. 17–23.

19. *Ibid.*

20. *Ibid.*, p. 66.

21. On this see Walter Burghardt, *Toward Reconciliation* (Washington: United States Catholic Conference, 1974).

22. On this see the article of Rahner cited earlier.

23. On this see the perceptive comments by Herbert McCabe O.P. in his *What Is Ethics All About?* (Washington: Corpus, 1969), pp. 91–92.

24. On this see Pius XII, "Address to Midwives," 26 Nov. 1951, in *Discorsi e Radio-messagi*, 13 (26 Nov. 1951): 415–417; see also *Acta Apostolicae Sedis*, 44 (1952): 416; cf. pp. 270–278.

25. There are, of course, great differences of opinion among contemporary Christian moralists about the way to determine the significance of human acts. Some, among them Joseph Fletcher, propose that the only way to do so is to do the loving thing, which means the deed that will help more people than it will hurt (cf. his *Situation Ethics* [Philadelphia: Westminster, 1965]). Fletcher's type of situation ethics is, as many writers have noted, a variant of utilitarianism and is a consequentialist approach to ethics. It is more interested in what our actions *get done* than in what they *get said*. For some excellent critiques of this approach see Germain Grisez, *Abortion: The Myths, The Realities, and the Arguments* (New York: Corpus, 1970), pp. 287–297; Paul Ramsey, *Deeds and Rules in Christian Ethics* (New York: Scribner's, 1967), chap. 7; and Stanley Hauerwas "Aslan and the New Morality," in his *Vision and Virtue* (South Bend: Fides, 1974). Many other contemporary moralists, in particular some Roman Catholic moral theologians, adopt a modified type of consequentialism, which can be called an ethics of the proportionate good. These authors hold that one can rightfully do and *intend to do* evil (e.g., kill a person or destroy his physical integrity) so long as there is a proportionate reason. The best statement of this position is by Richard McCormick in his *Ambiguity in Moral Choice* (Milwaukee: Marquette University Press, 1973). I have criticized this position in chapter 4 of my *Becoming Human: An Invitation to Christian Ethics* (Dayton: Pflaum, 1975) and in an article, "Ethics and Human Identity: The Challenge of the New Biology," *Horizons*, 3 (Spring 1976): 17–37. Grisez and Ramsey also have criticized this qualitative kind of consequentialism.

26. For a deeper discussion of the issues entailed see the works cited in note 25.

27. Grisez has developed his position in several places. The most

important works to consult are *Contraception and the Natural Law* (Milwaukee: Bruce, 1964), chap. 3; *Abortion: The Myths, the Realities and the Arguments* (New York: Corpus, 1970), chap. 6; and *Beyond the New Morality* (with Russell Shaw) (Notre Dame, Ind.: University of Notre Dame Press, 1974).

28. On this point see Mortimer Adler, *The Time of Our Lives* (New York: Holt, Rinehart and Winston, 1970), chap. 19.

29. See Grisez, *Contraception,* pp. 60–69, and *Abortion,* pp. 312–316.

30. On this see my essay, "The Natural Law, Conscience, and the Natural Law," *Communio,* 2 (Spring 1975) 3–32.

31. See *Summa Theologiae,* 1–2, 94, 2; Grisez, *Contraception,* pp. 60–66, and *Abortion,* pp. 312–316. See also the author's essay, "The Meaning and Nature of the Natural Law in Thomas Aquinas," *American Journal of Jurisprudence,* vol. 22 (1977).

32. *Ibid.*

33. *Ibid.*

34. Here we are touching on the meaning to be given to the rule or principle of double effect. For an understanding of this principle see Grisez, *Abortion,* pp. 321–334. A brief description of this principle is provided in my article, "Double Effect, Principle of," in *Encyclopedia of Bioethics,* ed. Warren Reich (New York: Macmillan–Free Press, 1978).

1: Experimenting on Human Subjects

In May 1973 a special CBS report, *The Ultimate Experimental Animal: Man,* telecast a scene that struck me as particularly illuminating, and it will introduce the question of experimenting on human beings. A black woman, who had been a prisoner in a Detroit jail, had participated in a program testing a new type of birth control pill. This particular pill was known to the researchers to carry a high risk of causing cancer, but this fact was not made known to the women who had "volunteered" to participate in the program testing its effectiveness. When the woman learned, after her release from prison, that the pill she and other women had been taking posed a serious risk of inducing cancer, she was outraged at having been "used," declaring to the CBS correspondent that she had been treated like an "animal."

Her reaction is quite instructive. In saying that she had been treated like an animal and in being outraged at having been so treated, she voiced the conviction that human beings ought not be treated like animals. She was not necessarily denying that she—and other human beings as well—is an animal (for, after all, we are) ; rather, she was affirming that a human being is an *animal with a difference,* the kind of being described in the Introduction as an entity of moral worth, a subject of rights that demand respect and protection from the society in which he or she lives. She was stating, in a simple and unsophisticated way, what Roger Wertheimer, a philosopher, has called a "standard belief" among human beings in our society. This is the belief that "being human has moral cachet; a human being has human status in virtue of being a human being,"[1] that being a member of the human species is a morally significant fact.[2]

She was, moreover, affirming that any experiment performed on the "human animal" must, if it is to be rightfully carried out, respect the fact that human beings are indeed entities of moral worth, subjects of rights that are rooted in their being and are not conferred upon them by others. She was affirming, at least implicitly, that no human being can be regarded simply as a part subordinated to a greater whole, the society at large, but must be considered as a whole that cannot rightfully be subordinated to the interests of others.

This is the cardinal point to be kept in mind as we consider the ethics of experimenting on human subjects. The moral worth of every human being is *the* crucial truth in considering this important topic. That every human being is a being of moral worth is central to the gospel and is eloquently proclaimed by the Church.[3] It is this truth alone that renders intelligible the cardinal principle in human experimentation, namely, the principle of free and informed consent, that "canon of loyalty," as Paul Ramsey terms it, which is operative in all situations wherein one human being is the experimenter and another is his "co-adventurer" in the experiment.[4] Before we look into this principle and its meaning, however, it is necessary to distinguish different types of experimental situations.

There are many types of experimental situations, but for our purposes they can be reduced to two general kinds: *therapeutic* and *nontherapeutic* or *research* experiments. Among the first can be included those experiments whose purpose is to (1) diagnose an illness from which a person is suffering, (2) alleviate or cure a malady from which the subject is suffering, and (3) prevent a person from becoming afflicted with a specifiable malady. Therapeutic experiments, in short, can be diagnostic, curative or alleviatory, or preventive. Despite the differences in these divergent therapeutic experiments, all are aimed at being of medical benefit to the subject.

Nontherapeutic or research experiments are not, of themselves, designed to be of medical benefit to the subject. Rather, they are intended to further biomedical and behavioral research, to advance the frontiers of knowledge and thus enable us to develop new techniques for coping with the diverse maladies that afflict mankind, and to enhance the human good. It is true that at times the subjects of such experiments may be benefited in a spiritual or psychological way,[5] but such a benefit to the subject is incidental to the experiment as such, inasmuch as it is aimed at benefiting persons other than the subject, whereas the therapeutic experiment is aimed at benefiting the subject.

There are "borderline" experiments, intended both to further knowledge (and thereby to benefit persons other than the experimental subject) and to benefit the subject. In attempting to develop a new flu vaccine, for instance, its use on a pilot group would be both therapeutic and research in intent. From the perspective of the ethical issues involved, centering around the principle of free and informed consent, such "experimentally" therapeutic experiments are to be classified with the therapeutic type.

The canon of loyalty that must be observed in *all* experimental situations, whether of the therapeutic or nontherapeutic or research type, is the principle of free and informed consent. This principle is at the heart of all medical ethics. It has been eloquently expressed in the articles of the Nuremberg Code (1946–1949), and it is important to recall that this code was formulated when the memory of the atrocities carried out by the Third Reich in the name of scientific research was fresh in the minds of men. According to the first article of the Nuremberg Code,

> The voluntary consent of the human subject is absolutely essential. This means that the person involved should have legal capacity to give consent; should be so situated as to be able to exercise free power of choice, without the intervention of any element of force, fraud, deceit, duress, overreaching, or other ulterior form of constraint or coercion; and should have sufficient knowledge and comprehension of the elements of the subject matter involved as to enable him to make an understanding and enlightened decision. This latter element requires that before the acceptance of an affirmative decision by the experimental subject there should be made known to him the nature, duration, and purpose of the experiment; the method and means by which it is to be conducted; all the

> inconveniences and hazards reasonably to be expected;
> and the effects upon his health or person which may pos-
> sibly come from his participation in the experiments.[6]

This concern that a human being who is to be the subject of an experiment give his free and informed consent is also reflected in the codes adopted by the World Health Organization in the *Declaration of Helsinki* in 1964,[7] by the American Medical Association in its 1966 convention,[8] and in the *Ethical and Religious Directives for Catholic Hospitals,* set forth in 1955 and revised in 1971.[9] This principle, at the heart of traditional Jewish and Christian medical ethics, has been reaffirmed again and again by the magisterium of the Roman Catholic Church.[10]

Many authorities, among them Henry K. Beecher, have noted that it is extremely difficult, if not impossible, to secure fully free and informed consent.[11] They have observed that frequently it is not possible to explain to the person about to undergo an experiment all of the factors involved. At times, the hazards may be unknown; at other times the persons who are to be the experimental subjects may not be capable of grasping all the pertinent and known factors; and at other times disclosure of all possible hazards might so terrify a person that he or she may not be willing to submit to an experiment that is really not hazardous and that offers reasonable hope of being beneficial. It is for such reasons that the American Medical Association, in commenting on the need for free and informed consent, saw fit to add that "in exceptional circumstances and to the extent that disclosure of information concerning the nature of the drug or experimental procedure or risks would be expected to materially affect the health of the patient and would be detrimental to his best interests, such information may be withheld from the patient."[12]

This means that the requirement or canon of loyalty, demanding free and informed consent, must be understood as demanding "reasonably" free and "adequately" informed consent, and the reasonableness and adequacy are to be determined as a prudent person would determine them. Ramsey puts it this way: "A choice may be free and responsible despite the fact that it began in an emotional bias one way or another, and consent can be informed without being encyclopedic."[13] Indeed, as Beecher notes repeatedly, the very fact that a sick person goes to a physician is an indication that he is giving reasonably free and informed consent to the physician's efforts to discover what is troubling him and to cure or alleviate the pathology.[14]

The requirement for reasonably free and adequately informed consent is essential in *all* types of human experimentation. The reason is simply that every human being, by being a member of the human species, is a being of moral worth, with rights that demand recognition, respect, and protection. Since every human being is of incomparable worth, with inherent dignity and value that transcend the society in which he or she lives,[15] each human being has the right to be regarded as one who cannot rightfully be *subordinated* to that society or to any person within it. Human beings are ends, not means, and all human beings are equal in their humanity.[16] Thus, as Ramsey says, "no man is good enough to experiment upon another without his consent."[17] To experiment on a human subject without securing his consent is to treat him as a being who is no longer of moral worth; to make of him a means, not an end; to subordinate him to other humans; to repudiate his humanity.

Proxy Consent

Yet there are instances, by no means rare, when it is impossible to obtain adequately informed and free consent from the person who is to be the subject of an experiment. What can be done—what *ought* to be done—when the subject, whether by reason of age, mental infirmity, or physical condition, is incapable of giving consent in his or her own behalf?

There is no serious debate among authorities, medical, legal, or moral, when the experiment in question is therapeutic, that is, when it is designed to secure some benefit for the subject. In cases of this kind, consent to the experiment can be given by others (parents, guardians, etc.) on behalf of persons incapable of giving consent for themselves. Writers speak in this connection of "proxy" or "presumptive" or "vicarious" consent, and there is unanimity that in therapeutic situations such proxy consent is morally justifiable.

There is serious debate, however, particularly among moral authorities, about proxy consent in the nontherapeutic situation. By examining this debate we can learn much about the significance of the principle of informed and free consent and can appreciate even more clearly why proxy consent is justifiable in the therapeutic situation.

Richard A. McCormick, the Jesuit moral theologian (currently serving as the Rose F. Kennedy Professor of Christian Ethics at the Center for Bioethics of the Kennedy Institute of Georgetown University), has pointed out that there are "two identifiable schools of (moral) thought [concerning this question]. . . . The first is associated with Paul Ramsey and is supported by William E. May. The second is the position of [Charles] Curran, [Thomas] O'Donnell, and myself."[18] To clarify this debate, in the belief that by doing so the deeply significant human values at stake will also be clarified, I propose to:

1. Outline the position taken by Ramsey early in the debate.

2. Summarize the position advanced by McCormick.

3. Note the objections I originally raised concerning this position.

4. Look at the reply given to these objections by McCormick.

5. Present some new reflections.

In his *Patient as Person,* Ramsey noted that some forms of non-therapeutic experimentation might not "harm" a child (or other human subject incapable of giving consent). Yet he argued that nontherapeutic experiments, that is, experiments designed not for the benefit of the subject but for the advancement of scientific knowledge and the benefit of persons other than the experimental subject,[19] constitute "offensive touching" and thus "wrong" the subject.[20] Developing his position, Ramsey wrote as follows:

> To attempt to consent for a child to be made an experimental subject is to treat a child as not a child. It is to treat him as if he were an adult person who has consented to become a joint adventurer in the common cause of medical research. If the grounds for this are alleged to be the presumptive or implied consent of the child, this must simply be characterized as a violent and a false presump-

tion. Nontherapeutic, non-diagnostic experimentation involving human subjects must be based on true consent if it is to proceed as a human enterprise. No child or adult incompetent can choose to become a participating member of medical undertakings, and no one else on earth should decide to subject these people to investigations having no relation to their own treatment. That is a canon of loyalty to them. This they claim of us simply by being a human child or incompetent. When he is grown, the child may put away childish things and become a true volunteer. This is the meaning of being a volunteer; that a man enter and establish a consensual relation in some joint venture for medical progress.[21]

In *Patient as Person* Ramsey also observed that when we use the term "proxy consent" to designate the human act in decisions to authorize therapeutic experiments on children and incompetent adults, the "consent" is in some degree a "false" consent. He noted that to construe or presume consent in such cases, we are by no means doing violence to the human being in whose behalf the consent is given, but he insisted that there is a degree of falsehood in using this expression.[22] His intent, I believe, was that it is simply false to say that a child or incompetent adult is "consenting" to the therapeutic experiment.

In his original essay, "Proxy Consent in the Experimental Situation," McCormick surprisingly did *not* develop a position that would seem to be in accord with his general moral theory, according to which the ultimate determinant of the rightness or wrongness of the deed in conflict situations is the proportionate or "higher" good that the deed is capable of achieving. (In this view, I believe, it would be relatively easy to develop a case for proxy consent in the nontherapeutic or experimental situation, based on the higher good that such experiments could achieve.)[23] Rather, he first sought to find the ultimate justification of proxy consent in the therapeutic situation in the moral theory sketched in the Introduction and developed by such contemporary philosophers and theologians as J. de Finance, G. de Broglie, G. Grisez, and John Finnis. Appealing to this theory, McCormick then sought to justify proxy consent not only in the therapeutic situation but in certain types of nontherapeutic or experimental situations.

The heart of his argument, as he himself restated it, is as follows:

> If we analyze proxy consent where it is accepted as legitimate—scil. in the *therapeutic* situation—we will see that parental consent is morally legitimate because, life and health being goods of the child, he would choose them because he *ought* to choose the good of life. In other words, proxy consent in the therapeutic situation is morally valid precisely insofar as it is a reasonable presumption of the child's wishes, a construction of what the child would wish could he do so. The child would so choose because he *ought* to do so, life and health being goods definitive of his flourishing.[24]

McCormick thus sees the ultimate justification of proxy consent in the therapeutic situation in the reasonableness of the presumption that the child or other incompetent would consent to the experiment if he could, and that he *would* consent because he *ought* to.

McCormick then applies this reasoning to the nontherapeutic or research or experimental situation. He is at pains to reject any "utilitarian evaluation of children's lives that would submit their integrity to a quantity-of-benefits calculus far beyond any legitimately constructed consent."[25] Yet he holds that there might be some types of nontherapeutic situations in which the consent of the child or other incompetent could be reasonably presumed, *if* one accepts the analysis he has provided of the rationale behind justifiable proxy consent in the therapeutic situation. His position, as recently summarized by McCormick himself, is expressed in this way:

> Once proxy consent in the therapeutic situation is analyzed in this way, the question occurs: are there other things that the child *ought,* as a human being, to choose precisely because and insofar as they are goods definitive of his well-being? As an answer to this question I have suggested that there are things we *ought* to do for others simply because we are members of the human community. These are not precisely works of charity or supererogation (beyond what is required of all of us) but our personal bearing of our share that all may prosper. They involve no discernible risk, discomfort or inconvenience, yet promise genuine hope for general benefit. In summary,

if it can be argued that it is a good for all of us to share
in these experiments, and hence that we *ought* to do so
(social justice), then a presumption of consent where
children are involved is reasonable, and proxy consent becomes legitimate.[26]

This argument proposes, therefore, that all of us have moral
obligations as members of the human community to contribute
our share to the "general benefit," that is, the common good,
when doing so entails no "discernible risk, discomfort, or incon-
venience." Because children and other incompetents are members of the human community, one can reasonably presume that
they would of themselves, if they could, choose to participate in
nontherapeutic experiments precisely because the child or other
incompetent "*ought* to want this not because it is in any way for
his own medical good, but because it is not (a) in any realistic
way to his harm and (b) represents a potentially great benefit to
others."[27]

It is very important to note that McCormick's justification of
proxy consent to nontherapeutic experiments on children and
other incompetents that involve no discernible or only minimal
risk[28] is inherently dependent for its validity on his analysis of
the rationale that justifies proxy consent in the therapeutic situation. I sought to stress this point in an earlier critique of Mc-
Cormick's position.[29] With Ramsey, I believe that the term "consent," when applied to instances when others give consent to an
experiment on a human being who is incapable of giving consent,
is in some degree falsely or improperly used. I therefore argued
that the justification of proxy consent in the therapeutic situation
in no way requires us to "construct" the consent of the child or
other incompetent by attempting to infer that he would, if he
could, consent to the experiment precisely because he *ought* to
do so if he is to manifest the love for the good of life and health
that is morally demanded of human subjects. Rather, I argued
that the basic justification for proxy consent in the therapeutic
situation is grounded in the moral obligations incumbent on parents and other adult members of the human community to do
what they can to protect the real goods of life and health when
these goods are imperiled in human beings who are incapable of

protecting these goods in themselves. In articulating my justification for proxy consent in the therapeutic situation I appealed to the Kew Gardens principle, as set forth by John Simon, Charles Powers, and Jon Gunnemann in their *The Ethical Investor*.[30] According to this principle, we (i.e., responsible adult human beings who are, properly speaking, moral beings or moral agents) have an obligation to do something in behalf of our fellow human beings when they are in need of help, when we are aware of the peril they are in (proximity), when we have some capacity for assisting them in their need (capability), and when they will surely suffer or be deprived of some basic human good if we do not take effective action (last resort).[31]

I should note that I could and perhaps should have appealed to the "'deontological" type of natural law theory defended by the writers to whom McCormick refers—the type sketched briefly in the Introduction—in order to justify proxy consent in the therapeutic situation, particularly since this was the theory to which McCormick had recourse in developing his position. It is important to look more closely at this theory and the way it ought, in my judgment, to be applied to the issue of proxy consent in both the therapeutic and the nontherapeutic situation.

According to the moral theory of the writers to whom McCormick appeals, the human good is pluriform, that is, it consists of a set of real goods that are constitutive of what can be called the whole or total human good, and these goods are real and not merely apparent because they are inherently related to real needs that are rooted in our being. Among these goods are life and health. Neither life nor health nor any of the basic human goods is, as we have seen, the supreme good or *summum bonum*, but each is a real good of real human beings and each, *as known*, functions as a principle of practical reason, or what we could call a principle of intelligent human behavior.[32]

There are several ways, according to this theory, in which the basic human goods that give rise to affirmative moral principles bind us. In his articulation of this theory Grisez distinguishes five modes of obligation. I shall note them here and simply point out that his third mode is precisely the mode of obligation involved in what Simon, Gunneman, and Powers call the Kew Gardens principle and is, in my judgment, the operative mode in the therapeutic situation when the human subject is incapable of giving consent. According to Grisez, the basic modes of obligation are the following:

> In the first place, all of these goods bind us at least to this, that we take them into account. In our practical reasoning, we must have a permanent sensitivity to the essential goods to which primary principles direct. An attitude of simple disregard for any one of them reveals that we have set ourselves against it. Therefore, such an attitude is incompatible with our basic obligation to pursue good and to act for it.
>
> In the second place, every one of the goods demands of us that when we can do so as easily as not, we avoid acting in ways which inhibit its realization and prefer ways of acting which contribute to its realization. This principle can never be applied legalistically, but nevertheless its use is quite common in practice in ordinary moral arguments.
>
> . . . In the third place, every one of the goods demands of us that we make an effort on its behalf when its significant realization in some person is in extreme peril. This obligation frequently binds with great force. . . . This type of obligation binds in degrees varying with the seriousness of the stake, the immediacy of the peril, and the opportunity we and others have for giving aid. . . .
>
> In the fourth place, every one of the goods demands of us that we do not act directly against its realization. . . .
>
> Still another, the fifth way, in which the values establish obligations is that each of them demands that we keep our engagements with it. We do not have a general obligation to seek out opportunities for promoting every one of the goods. But we should pursue some good, and each person according to his individual aptitude must choose the values he will try to promote.[33]

It should be obvious that the third mode of obligation is at stake when so-called proxy consent is given in the therapeutic situation. It is simply a way of stating the Kew Gardens principle in the language of the moral theory to which McCormick appealed in articulating his position.

If this is true, then the basic reason why it is morally legitimate for a parent or other adult to consent to allow his child or other incompetent human being to participate in a therapeutic experiment is simply that the consent in such cases is an exercise of proper moral responsibility by a moral agent of the obligation he has to promote the good of another human being when this good is imperiled and when the former has the capacity of defending and protecting it. There is no need for him to construct the child's wishes or to presume that the child would of himself consent to the procedure, if he could, because of any moral obligation on his part to do so. In a similar way, a responsible moral agent would consent to a therapeutic experiment on a dog or cat.

My original objection to the position of McCormick was based on the belief that his analysis of the justification of proxy consent in the therapeutic situation is inaccurate and that, *a fortiori,* his analysis of such justification in the nontherapeutic situation is erroneous. I claimed that his position requires one to treat a child or other incompetent human subject as a moral agent, something that a child or other incompetent, simply by being a child or incompetent, certainly is not.[34] I then argued that in the nontherapeutic situation it would be wrong for a parent or other adult to consent for a child or other incompetent human subject. In such instances the child or other incompetent human subject is in no need; no basic human good is imperiled. Nor does the child or other incompetent have a moral obligation to the general benefit or common good, precisely because they are not moral agents and hence do not bear any moral responsibilities or moral obligations. But a child or other incompetent human subject *is* a being of moral worth, a subject of inviolable rights, and adult members of the human community who *are* moral agents and bearers of moral obligations must respect him as such. To "volunteer" the child for an experiment that is of no benefit to him is to violate this respect, for it is to treat him not as a child, a being of moral worth who has no moral obligations, but as an adult, a being of moral worth who has moral obligations. It is, in other words, to refuse to recognize him for what he is and to consider him as being what he is not.

Commenting on these objections, McCormick made two points. His first point was that the position he originally advanced did not "necessarily regard the infant as a moral agent. Nor need it [he wrote] imply that he has obligations. It need only suggest that what it is reasonable and legitimate to do experimentally with youngsters might be constructed off what others who are moral agents *ought* as humans to do; for though they are not yet moral agents, infants are humans in the fullest sense."[35]

Note that in replying to the objections McCormick now says that his position does not necessarily imply that an infant has moral obligations. His present contention that this is not implied by his analysis does not seem to me to be a proper reply. For he not only implied that the infant has moral obligations but *asserted explicitly* that this was the case. For he wrote: "Proxy consent is morally valid precisely insofar as it is a reasonable presumption of *the child's wishes,* a construction of what the child would wish could he do so. The child would so choose because he *ought* to do so."[36] If this is not to presume or infer or construct moral obligations in the child, I have difficulty grasping what it is.

With respect to McCormick's claim that his position "need only suggest that what is reasonable and legitimate to do experimentally with youngsters might be constructed off what others who are moral agents *ought* as humans to do; for though they are not yet moral agents, infants are humans in the fullest sense," the following observations are in order.

With McCormick, I believe that infants and adult incompetents are humans in the fullest sense, but I believe that we need to make distinctions when we speak of what *we as humans ought to do.* I believe that I do not, precisely *as* a human being, a member of the human species, have *any* moral obligations. Yet I believe that I am, precisely as a member of the human species, a being of moral worth, an image of God. As a human being, I am radically capable of *becoming* a moral agent, a being with moral obligations, but in order to become such an entity I need the help of the human community. In reflecting on why this is so we will be led, I believe, to a deeper insight into the moral values in the issue of proxy consent and why such consent is not justifiable in the nontherapeutic situation.

No one who reads these lines—no human being anywhere—was a moral being or moral agent at birth. No one who reads these lines—no human being anywhere—was a person or personal subject at birth, if by *person* or *personal subject* one means a self-conscious entity who is aware of itself as a self, as an enduring subject of experience, capable of communicating with other persons, other selves, and capable of distinguishing between *is* and *ought,* of recognizing the basic human goods and of loving them and the persons in whom they are incarnated. Empirical evidence is revealing here, such as instances of feral or "wolf" children, that is, human infants, separated from a human community quite early in their lives, who were reared by animals such as wolves or bears. When these human offspring—beings *certainly* human by reason of their membership in the human species and, in my judgment (and, I believe, in Christian faith), infinitely precious beings imaging the living God—were found by other human beings and brought back into the human community, it was evident that they had no realization or awareness of themselves as selves. They totally lacked the concept of selfhood; indeed, they were incapable of entertaining *any* concepts. They were, in brief, quite innocent of their identity as human beings and were in no way bearers of moral obligations.

This fact makes us acutely aware of the social solidarity of our existence as human beings. It shows us that human existence, as personal existence, is inescapably and necessarily co-existence, or that, to use a biblical expression, human existence is *covenantal in character.* To be human, in the sense that "to be human" means being personal and being a self who is aware of his responsibilities, is to exist *with* other human beings. But for us to exist *with* other human beings, we must first be granted leave by them to exist with them. Personhood, in other words, is a gift. It is, in a very real sense and in one respect, a gift that each of us receives from other human beings, although ultimately God is the source of our personhood. It is a gift we receive, directly and immediately, from the parents who conceived us, in an act that was, at the same time, one hopes, expressive of the love they had for one another, and it is a gift that we are continually called upon to bestow on one another. My being me depends, in a very real way, on your being you and allowing me to be me. An indispensable prerequisite for our becoming persons is the help of the human community. We must first be recognized by that community for what we are, namely, beings of moral worth, if we are to be enabled to grow into personhood.

Perhaps I can express this more clearly if I reformulate the strikingly perceptive formulation of the Golden Rule suggested by Roger Wertheimer in the essay that was cited at the beginning of this chapter. I submit the following: You, a moral being (i.e., a personal subject, capable of rational reflection, of exercising moral responsibility, and of being the bearer of moral obligations), are to do unto others (i.e., other members of the human species, other beings of moral worth) as you, a member of the human species and a being of moral worth, would have others (i.e., other moral beings, other personal subjects who are capable of rational reflection, of exercising moral responsibility, and of being the bearers of moral obligations) do unto you, a member of the human species, a being of moral worth.

Apply this now to the instances when proxy consent is at issue. In the therapeutic situation, human beings who have become moral agents and bearers of moral obligations (because they have at least been allowed to be and have been in some way recognized for what they really are by the human community) face a moral obligation to do what they rightly can do to help a fellow human being (a being of moral worth) participate in the true human goods of health and life. In the nontherapeutic situation, the same human beings are required to recognize in an infant or other incompetent human subject the reality that is present to them and demand that they recognize him as the entity he really is. To authorize that this human being be made to participate in an experiment that is in no way related to his well-being and in which he is required to participate simply because he can provide an indispensable ingredient for the success of the experiment is an act, I submit, that ruptures the covenantal bonds that ought to exist in and among human beings, for it is to regard this human subject, this being of moral worth, either as an impersonal "it" or as a bearer of moral obligations, neither of which he is. This is a point that has now been stressed quite forcefully by Ramsey.[37]

To put it another way, I believe that proxy consent in nontherapeutic situations is morally unjustifiable precisely because it strikes at the very heart of the belief or presupposition that makes the principle of free and informed consent intelligible and true to begin with, namely, that all human beings, simply by reason of their membership in the human species, are beings of moral worth and, as such, entities that transcend the communities in which they live.

The second point McCormick raises in commenting on the earlier criticism of his position is: "At some point the discussion must come to grips with the fact that Ramsey's position ('offensive touching') —the one preferred by May—could not allow any non-therapeutic experimentation whatsoever, even the most trivial such as a buccal smear or routine weighing."[38] What about this?

A buccal smear, as I understand it, is tissue taken from human cheeks for examination. I do not know whether buccal smears are routinely done on infants, but, if so, I believe one ought seriously to question the practice, unless it is done to help or in some way benefit the infants whose cheek tissue is used for examination. Similarly, if the weighing of infants is in no way related to their well-being, the act ought not be performed. Surely any of us—and I imagine that McCormick would be included—would be "offended," and rightly so, if someone were to take tissue from our cheeks or put us on a scale simply out of curiosity and without asking our leave. It would be an affront to our dignity, to our humanity. Since infants are, as McCormick admits, human in the fullest sense, are they not offensively touched when buccal smears and weighings, in no way related to their well-being, are done? The "inoffensiveness" of such deeds exists only in the minds of those responsible for such acts, and is the result of their insensitivity.

Quite recently McCormick has, in further responding to criticisms made by Ramsey and me about his position, stated that his original position was predicated not so much on imputed moral obligations in the child but rather on the sociability of the child. His point seems to be that the child must be regarded not as an isolated individual but as a member of a community, and as a member of the community the child can reasonably be expected to contribute to the common good of the community. At times this contribution could be by participating in nontherapeutic experimentations that carry no discernible or only minimal risk and that can be of great value to the entire community. He then claims that the position taken by Ramsey and me is too "individualistic," one that fails to take seriously into account the social character of all human life, including the life of children.[39]

McCormick is quite correct in insisting on the corporate, social character of our existence as human beings. In fact, I would prefer to refer to this as the *covenantal* dimension of our being. But there is a vast difference between the way this dimension of our existence is expressed in a child and in an adult. An adult is aware of the social, corporate character of his existence. He is conscious of the obligations that he has to others, of the demand that he recognize them for who they are and respond to their needs. An adult is, by definition, a morally responsible agent, aware of his social nature and of his obligation to contribute to the common good. A child is as yet not aware of his social obligations. His sociability consists in his need and right to be cared for by others and to arrive, with their help, at an understanding of himself and his responsibilities as a social being. But until he arrives at this understanding he is incapable of contributing to the common good *by his actions,* inasmuch as he simply cannot engage in human actions as a child, as one who is not aware of his responsibilities and who is not capable of determining his life through his own free choices. As a child he contributes to the common good just by being. The adults in the community owe him the obligation to recognize him for who he is, namely a child who needs help to develop his capacities so that he can become an adult. They need to have a reverence for his integrity and inviolability, his being as a being of moral worth. And they violate this integrity and inviolability by touching him offensively, by "volunteering" him for actions that in and of themselves require personal consent, that require a genuine volunteer.

I realize that the position set forth in this chapter in many ways restricts what medical researchers can rightfully do to develop new technologies that will be of benefit to the human race. Such restrictions, however, flow from love for the inherent worth of each human being and are demanded by this love and respect. To touch human beings offensively by "volunteering" them for an adventure in which they cannot, by reason of their condition, be volunteers is to attack not simply them but the dignity of *all* human beings.

In drawing these comments to a close, it is fitting, I believe, to draw attention to the views of three writers, each working from a different perspective, who have thought seriously and deeply about human experimentation: Henry Beecher, the medical scientist; Hans Jonas, the philosopher; and Pius XII, the universal teacher. For Beecher, an experiment on a human subject does not *become* morally right because it succeeds in its purposes; rather, it must be morally right from its very inception.[40] According to Jonas, we ought not be overly concerned about what society can "afford" in the way of losing precious experimental materials; rather, we should be very concerned about what a really human society *cannot* afford, namely, "a single miscarriage of justice, a single inequity in the dispensation of its laws, the violation of the rights of even the tiniest minority, because these undermine the moral basis on which the society's existence rests."[41] For Pius XII, the moral history of mankind is more important than its scientific history.[42]

If we take seriously the truths these thoughtful persons have expressed, we realize that there may be some things that we can come to know, and that would be good for us to know, but that the very endeavor to gain knowledge of them is impossible without doing something that we, as moral agents, ought not do.

Chapter 1

1. Roger Wertheimer, "Philosophy on Humanity," in Robert L. Perkins, ed., *Abortion: Pro and Con* (Cambridge, Mass.: Schenkmann, 1975), pp. 107–128 at pp. 107–108.

2. That membership in the human species is a morally significant fact is denied by those who, with Michael Tooley and Joseph Fletcher, distinguish between being a human being and being a person or "enduring subject of experiences, aware of itself as a self." Tooley explicitly denies that membership in the human species is itself morally significant, and this denial is implicit in the thought of Fletcher and many other contemporary writers. See Michael Tooley, "Abortion and Infanticide," *Philosophy and Public Affairs,* 3 (Fall 1972): 37–65, and Joseph Fletcher, "Indicators of Humanhood," *Hastings Center Report,* 2 (November 1972): 1–4. For a critique of this view see my "What Makes a Human Being to Be a Being of Moral Worth?" *The Thomist,* 40 (July, 1976): 416–443.

3. See, e.g., *Gaudium et Spes,* par. 19.

4. Paul Ramsey, *The Patient as Person* (New Haven: Yale University Press, 1970), p. 5.

5. There is a tendency in some writers, e.g., Martin Nolan, to justify some kinds of activities in terms of a spiritual or moral good that will be secured by a person willing to undergo an experiment. This is a view that Ramsey terms the "sticky benefits" theory. See Nolan's essay, "The Principle of Totality," in Charles E. Curran, ed., *Absolutes in Moral Theology?* (Washington: Corpus, 1968).

6. The Nuremberg Code, art. 1. Text is given in Henry K. Beecher, *Research and the Individual* (Boston: Little, Brown, 1970), p. 277.

7. The Helsinki Declaration, 1964, in Beecher, *op. cit.,* p. 227.

8. AMA Code, art. 1, i, in Beecher, *op. cit.,* pp. 221f.

9. *Ethical and Religious Directives for Catholic Hospitals.* The text of the 1955 statement is given in Beecher, *op. cit.,* p. 245. The text of the 1971 statement is available from the Catholic Hospital Association and is provided in the appendix of John Dedek, *Contemporary Medical Ethics* (New York: Sheed and Ward, 1975).

10. See the numerous statements of Pius XII on this subject, gathered in *The Pope Speaks,* vol. 1, nos. 3 and 4 (1954). Among the principal addresses by Pius XII on this subject are those to the First International Congress on the Histopathology of the Nervous System (Sept. 14, 1952), the Sixteenth International Congress of Military Medicine (Oct. 19, 1953), and his address to the Eighth Congress of the World Medical Association (Sept. 30, 1954).

11. Beecher, *op. cit.,* pp. 18–19, 121ff., passim.

12. AMA Code, art. 3, i, in Beecher, *op. cit.,* p. 222.

13. Ramsey, *op. cit.,* p. 3.

14. Beecher, *op. cit.,* pp. 18–19, 231f.

15. On this point see Jacques Maritain, *The Person and the Common Good* (New York: Scribner's, 1947), chap. 3.

16. This truth is well developed by Mortimer Adler in his *The Difference of Man and the Difference It Makes* (New York: Meridian, 1968).

17. Ramsey, *op. cit.,* p. 7.

18. Richard A. McCormick, "Fetal Research, Morality, and Public Policy," a paper prepared for the National Commission for the Protection of Human Subjects of Biomedical and Behavioral Research and printed in *Hastings Center Report,* 5 (June 1975): 27.

19. On this notion of nontherapeutic experimentation see LeRoy Walters, "Fetal Research and the Ethical Issues," another paper pre-

pared for the commission and found in *Hastings Center Report,* 5 (June 1975): 15.

20. Ramsey, *op. cit.,* pp. 27–40.

21. *Ibid.,* p. 14.

22. *Ibid.,* p. 11.

23. Richard A. McCormick, "Proxy Consent in the Experimental Situation," *Perspectives in Biology and Medicine* (Fall 1974). This essay was reprinted with minor changes in James Johnston and David Smith, eds., *Love and Society: Essays in the Ethics of Paul Ramsey* (Missoula, Mont.: Scholars' Press, 1974), pp. 209–228. It is from this latter source that citations are taken here.
McCormick's general moral theory, which was alluded to in note 25 of the Introduction, makes the notion of the "proportionate" or "greater" good sovereign in the moral domain. He articulates this theory most clearly in his *Ambiguity in Moral Choice* (Milwaukee: Marquette University Press [Pere Marquette Lecture in Theology], 1973), where he shows how it is discernible in the writings of many contemporary Roman Catholic moral theologians, among them Bruno Schüller, Cornelius Van der Poel, William Van der Marck, Louis Janssens, et al. In his essay McCormick acknowledges that his is a form of consequentialism. His basic argument is that one may properly intend evil (e.g., violation of the personal integrity of a subject of experimentation) so long as there is a proportionate or greater good to be gained. He holds that in such instances the evil is intended only in itself, not for itself, and that it is only when evil is intended both in and for itself that the act is wrong and the doer makes himself an evildoer. I have criticized this view extensively in my article "Ethics and Human Identity: The Challenge of the New Biology," in *Horizons: The Journal of the College Theology Society,* 3 (Spring 1976): 17–37. It should be noted that both Germain Grisez and Paul Ramsey, who develop a position along the lines suggested in the Introduction, have recently written very substantive critiques of this "proportionate good" type of consequentialism for an anthology that is soon to be published by Yale University Press. This position will be discussed at more length below, in chapter 2, pp. 59–61, and chapter 6, pp. 134–142.

24. McCormick, "Fetal Research, Morality, and Public Policy," *loc. cit.,* p. 27. McCormick restated his position in the same language in his "Notes on Moral Theology," *Theological Studies,* 36 (March 1975): 127.

25. McCormick, "Fetal Research, Morality, and Public Policy," p. 27.

26. *Ibid.* See also his "Notes on Moral Theology," 1975, p. 127.

27. McCormick, "Proxy Consent in the Experimental Situation," pp. 220–221.

28. McCormick's position seemingly provided the basis for the consensus of the National Commission for the Protection of Human Subjects of Biomedical and Behavioral Research. See, e.g., the essays by Peter Steinfels, LeRoy Walters, and Stephen Toulmin in the issue of *Hastings Center Report* referred to in notes 18 and 19 above.

29. See my article, "Experimenting on Human Subjects," *Linacre Quarterly*, 41 (November 1974): 238–252.

30. New Haven: Yale University Press (1972), pp. 22–25.

31. *Ibid.*

32. See Germain Grisez, *Contraception and the Natural Law* (Milwaukee: Bruce, 1964), chap. 3.

33. Grisez, *op. cit.,* pp. 84–86.

34. See my "Experimenting on Human Subjects," pp. 247–248.

35. McCormick, "Notes on Moral Theology," p. 128.

36. *Ibid.,* p. 127.

37. This thought is developed at length by Ramsey in his critique of McCormick, "The Enforcement of Morals: Nontherapeutic Experimentation on Children," *Hastings Center Report,* vol. 6 (May 1976).

38. McCormick, "Notes on Moral Theology," p. 128.

39. This objection was brought to my attention by readers of the article on experimentation (cited in n. 29) in private correspondence. This objection has since been articulated by McCormick in his response to the essay by Ramsey noted in n. 37. McCormick's response is found in *Hastings Center Report* 6 (October, 1976). It appeared after this chapter had been written, but in making the text ready for the printer I have at least been able to refer to his criticism and, in the text, to outline the type of answer that seems pertinent. It is quite important to note, however, that McCormick now seems to be basing his argument on the sociability of the child and not on a construction of the child's wishes and obligations. He has, in short, repudiated his original position and is now attempting a new argument based on the sociability of children.

40. H. K. Beecher, "Ethics and Clinical Research," *New England Journal of Medicine,* 274 (1966): 1354.

41. Hans Jonas, "Philosophical Reflections on Experimentations with Human Subjects," *Daedalus* (Spring, 1969).

42. Pius XII, "Address to the First International Congress on the Histopathology of the Nervous System" (Sept. 14, 1952), in *The Pope Speaks,* vol. 1, no. 3 (1954).

2: Beginning Human Life: Procreating or Reproducing?

New ways of initiating human life have been made possible by developments in scientific knowledge and technology. Some of these are already available and are being used, for example, artificial insemination, either by husband or donor, whereas others are being developed and may become available either in the immediate future—for instance, *in vitro* fertilization, with subsequent implantation of the developing embryo in the womb of the mother, the womb of a "surrogate" mother, or an artificial uterus—or in the remote future, for instance, cloning. These new ways for beginning human life can all be considered forms of reproduction. Before we examine some of them and reflect on the questions they raise about their justifiable use, however, it is important to look at the "old" (and still quite current) way in which new human life commences in order to reflect on *its* significance. Although the old way is considered by some to be a form of reproduction, it can also be understood, and in my judgment is better understood, as an act of procreation.

Sex: Life Giving and Love Giving

From the time that man first emerged on earth until the very recent past, new human beings came into existence through the sexual union of a man and a woman. The man was the father of the child who was brought into being through this union, and the woman was its mother. This same phenomenon—the generation of new life through the sexual union of male and female—is, of course, observable in many animal species. However, since the human animal is different in kind from other animals, there is reason to believe that this phenomenon has a significance for the human animal that it does not have for other animals. As evidence of this, there are strikingly significant features in human generation that are absent in animals of other species. In no other animal species, for example, can we observe such long postnatal fathering and such long-term relationships between the male and the female as in the human species.[1] In addition, in no other animal species is the child, generated by sexual union, so utterly helpless and dependent for such a prolonged period as in the human species. It is worth pondering these facts, seeking to discover their meaning.

An act of sexual intercourse between a man and a woman can, and frequently does, issue in the conception of a new human being. Such acts, of course, do not of necessity issue in a new human life, but their capacity to do so is meaningful and indicates that there is an inherent connection between human sexual intercourse and the beginning of a new human life. To put this another way, it can be said that there is a generative or *procreative,* that is, life-giving, potential or dimension to human sexual intercourse. Although this procreative dimension does not exhaust the intelligibility of human sexual intercourse, it is by no means accidental but is inherently meaningful.[2]

In addition to its procreative dimension, human sexual intercourse is capable of uniting a man and a woman in an intimate, personal union. Through acts of sexual intercourse a man and a woman can express their deep love for one another, their willingness to be with and for one another, their unity in one flesh, their communion in being. An act of sexual intercourse, in short, can be a special way in which a man and a woman share their lives, their selves. Sexual intercourse therefore has a *unitive,* that is, a love-giving, potential or dimension.

In the same act, moreover, a man and a woman can communicate their mutually shared life and love to a new human being, to a new generation. Thus the love that unites the woman and the man and is expressed in the act of sexual union includes not only themselves but reaches out to a new human life and will provide the "root room" in which that life can develop properly. It creates the conditions under which a new human being, of moral worth, will be wanted and given an opportunity to become fully what it is. The children who may be brought into being as a result of this kind of love will, in turn, deepen the union between the man and the woman; they will be living symbols of this union. There is, in other words, a unique interrelationship between the procreative or life-giving dimension of human sexual intercourse and its unitive or love-giving dimension. These two dimensions, though distinct and separable, are inherently interrelated. Each is meaningful and their meaningfulness is interpenetrating.

This surely tells us something about the meaning of human existence and the role, within human existence, of human sexual intercourse. Through sexual intercourse, as through all human acts, we reveal our identity; we tell people who we are and we discover who we are. At the same time, through our acts we shape our lives for the future, conferring an identity upon ourselves.

Through an act of sexual intercourse we can, of course, cut ourselves off from others, even from the other with whom we have intercourse, and thereby reveal our attitude toward life and the "goods" that make for a full human life. We show that we regard these goods as private possessions, to be pursued at our pleasure, and that we regard other human beings as objects to serve our needs. We thereby indicate that we think human life and its goods are not to be shared by all but are intended just for us. Or we can show, in intercourse, that we love human life and the goods of life precisely because they are human goods and are lovable because they are perfective of human beings, that they are meant to be shared with and communicated to other human beings, including those of a future generation.

Since sexual intercourse is a way of sharing life and love, and indeed of sharing them with a new generation, it is reasonable to infer that persons who have sexual intercourse should be capable of sharing life with one another. This means that they ought to have some kind of common past, a common or shared history, a life that goes beyond communication to issue in communion. In brief, they ought not be strangers. It also means that they ought to be committed to one another, that they be willing to face the future together, to risk their lives together, confident that the trust they put in one another will not be betrayed, or, if betrayed, that the wounds can be healed by a reconciling love. Human beings are the most vulnerable animals, and in giving themselves to one another in an act of sexual love they open themselves to the possibilities of a terrible wound; but the risk is warranted if the conditions for love and trust are present.

In addition, since the act of sexual union is capable of communicating life and love to a future generation, this possibility must be recognized for what it is, a good, a blessing, not a curse. There should be a readiness, unless special conditions are present, to give life to that generation and to care for that new life by providing it with the climate necessary for its nourishment and development; in short, for giving it a home. All this adds up to what is meant by marriage and a family.

Marriage is not a matter of legalistic ceremonies and juridical obligations, it is a covenantal relationship. It is a relationship in which a man and a woman pledge their lives to each other and pledge themselves to a future they do not know but are willing to enter together, to share with one another and with a new human generation.[3] It is a human reality that truly images and makes present the relationship between God and the entire community of mankind, precisely because God exists both with and for us and we, his living icons, are meant to exist with and for one another. It is thus a human reality that is fit to become and to be a *sacramentum*, a sacred reality that communicates God's love, life, and grace.

In saying all this I am not saying that human sexual intercourse is always an expression of love, an act of friendship and communion. I am saying that this is what human sexual intercourse, of its own finality and in accord with the providence of God, tends to be; it is what is meant to be and what it ought to be. It is also true that an act of sexual union is not necessarily generative of new human life. Still, its procreative potential is an inherently intelligible dimension and the relationship between this procreative meaning and the unitive meaning of sexual intercourse is inherently meaningful.

Since Paul Ramsey has clearly and vigorously articulated some cardinal ideas that are pertinent to the relationship between the procreative or life-giving and the unitive or love-giving aspects of human sexual intercourse, it will be helpful to cite him at some length.

> An act of sexual intercourse is at the same time an act of love and a procreative act. This does not mean that sexual intercourse always in fact nourishes love between the parties or always engenders a child. It simply means that it *tends,* of its own nature, toward the engendering of children (the procreative good), and toward the strengthening of love (the unitive or communicative good). This will be the nature of human sexual relations, provided there is no obstruction to the realization of these natural ends. . . . The crucial question is whether . . . sexual intercourse as an act of love should ever be separated from sexual intercourse as a procreative act. . . . Now I will state as a premise of the following discussion [of genetic control] that an ethics . . . that *in principle* severs these two goods—regarding procreation as an aspect of biological nature to be subjected merely to the requirements of *technical* control while saying that the unitive purpose is the free, human personal end of the matter—pays disrespect to the nature of human parenthood. . . . Most Protestants, and nowadays a great many Catholics, endorse contraceptive devices which separate the sex act as an act of love from whatever tendency there may be in the act (at the time of the act, and in the sexual powers of the parties) toward the engendering of a child. But they do *not* separate the sphere or realm of their procreation, nor do they distinguish between the *person* with whom the bond of love is nourished and the *person* with whom the procreation may be brought into exercise. One has only to distinguish what is done in particular *acts* from what is intended, and done, in a whole series of acts of conjugal intercourse in order to see clearly that contraception need not be a radical attack upon what God joined together in the creation of man–womanhood. Where planned parenthood is not planned *un*parenthood, the husband and wife clearly do not tear their own one-flesh unity completely away from all positive response and obedience to the mystery of procreation.[4]

Ramsey's statement not only summarizes much of what has

been said already, it raises other pertinent questions. He obviously endorses contraceptive intercourse if there are serious reasons
for avoiding conception, and in doing so he makes use of an argument that has been widely accepted by many Roman Catholic
moral theologians. This argument, in fact, is central to the rationale in the famous "majority report" of the Pontifical Commission on Population, Family, and Birth, more popularly known
as the Birth Control Commission.[5] In this view, the procreative
and unitive meanings or dimensions of human sexual intercourse
are inherently interrelated, and a marriage ought as such to be
open to procreation. This view, in other words, repudiates the
ideology of nonprocreative sex that is so common today and is
represented in the writings of such authors as Joseph Fletcher,[6]
Robert and Anna Francoeur,[7] Ashley Montagu,[8] and many others.
(This view, however, maintains that it is morally justifiable to
render specific acts of intercourse within the marital covenant
infertile by human intervention for serious reasons—which raises
a very serious question. Since, however, the practice of contraceptive intercourse will occupy our attention in this study primarily as a way of protecting the human genetic pool by preventing
the conception and birth of children who might be seriously
handicapped by genetically caused diseases, discussion of this
issue will be reserved for the next chapter, where I will seek to
show why contraceptive intercourse is not a morally justifiable
way of coping with this problem.) My principal reason for citing
Ramsey here is that he expresses, clearly and eloquently, human
values as they pertain especially to the *new* beginnings of human
life, made possible by biomedical advancements, and as we relate
these new ways of generating human life to procreation through
sexual union.

These new beginnings are all in some measure alternatives to
procreation, to the human act in which a man and a woman unite
in an act of sexual intercourse that is meant to be an expression
of their love and friendship and, *at the same time,* can communicate to a new human being the life and love they bear for one
another. These new beginnings, in some measure, separate the
unitive and procreative dimensions of human sexual intercourse.
They have, therefore, an impact on what George Gilder has called

the "sexual constitution of the species,"[9] and for this reason alone it is necessary to be very critical in evaluating these procedures.

There is something incomparably precious and deeply meaningful for our understanding of our lives together as human beings in the fact that a man and a woman can commit themselves fully to one another, giving and receiving one another in an act that makes them one and by which—*at the same time, in the very act that is so expressive of their love for one another**—they give life to

*It is imperative to recognize that sexual intercourse, although one of the most wonderful ways whereby a man and a woman can express their love for one another, is by no means the greatest or deepest expression of that love. The sacrificial love a spouse gives her husband or his wife in caring for her or him during sickness and in times of terrible suffering, when there is no possibility of intercourse, is an even greater manifestation of spousal love.

a new human being of moral worth, whom they are to receive and give a home, where he can take root and grow, discover himself, find his identity, and be given the opportunity to become fully the being he really is. The questions posed by Leon Kass are pertinent here, and their answers seem evident: "Is there possibly some wisdom in that mystery of nature which joints the pleasure of sex, the communication of love, and the desire for children in the very activity by which we continue the chain of human existence? Is biological parenthood a built-in 'device' selected to promote the adequate caring for posterity?"[10]

Proposed Methods of Reproduction

With these reflections on the meaning of sex as life giving and love giving and on the generation of human beings as an act of procreation, we can look at some of the alternatives to sexual union between a man and a woman that have been and are being proposed for the initiation of new human life. All of these proposals are clearly described by Gerald Leach in his informative book *The Biocrats*.[11] Major proposals include artificial insemination, either by husband or by donor, and at times with frozen sperm; test-tube or *in vitro* fertilization, with subsequent implantation of the embryo in the womb of the "biological" mother, or another woman, or possibly outside the human womb in an artificial uterus; embryo "banks," or the freezing of embryos who are brought into being either naturally or artificially, are selected by potential parents, and develop either *in utero* or outside; and cloning. The technologies are well described by Leach and many others, including Gordon Rattray Taylor[12] and Albert Rosenfeld,[13] and have been popularized in most of the major newsmagazines and cultural journals,[14] so that there is no necessity to describe them in any detail here.

Why are these alternatives to coital generation advocated? Artificial insemination by the husband or a donor, as currently practiced, and *in vitro* fertilization, as proposed by its leading advocates, are advanced as ways of fulfilling the desire of a woman for bearing her own child when such fulfillment is impeded by the husband's infertility, or low sperm count or other factors, or by blocked Fallopian tubes.[15] Artificial insemination by the husband, with sperm that was previously ejaculated and frozen, is also advocated as a way for a husband who must be away from spouse and family for long periods to "keep in touch," as it were, and is suggested as a type of "insurance" for men who undergo vasectomies in order to avoid conception, in the event that later they should choose to father a child. Also, donor artificial insemination or donor egg grafts, test-tube fertilization, sperm banks, and cloning, some believe, could be means for enhancing the quality of the human genetic pool, for raising the quality of life, and for producing the "optimum" baby. The eugenic purposes of these techniques will be discussed at more length in the next chapter. Here we will focus on artificial insemination, by husband and by donor, and test-tube fertilization as ways of fulfilling human desires.

Artificial Insemination by Husband (AIH)

Artificial insemination by the husband, also called homologous insemination, is not too common. Leach tells us that "the commonest reasons for it are malformed male organs, impotence, very low virility where intercourse is rare, or premature ejaculation. In other words, there are usually quite serious psycho-sexual disturbances in the marriage relationship."[16] If these are the reasons for resorting to AIH, most physicians, Leach observes, refuse to help.[17] Another main cause for AIH is gross male subfertility, and since this does not imply psychosexual difficulties between husband and wife, more physicians are willing to assist in the process.[18]

Until recently, most Roman Catholic moralists, following the lead of Pope Pius XII, rejected artificial insemination by the husband unless this could be rightly considered as "assisted natural insemination."[19] Pius himself, while condemning AIH if it entails procuring the sperm by "acts contrary to nature,"[20] had added that he was not necessarily proscribing "the use of certain artificial means designed only to facilitate the natural act or to enable that act, performed in a normal manner, to attain its end."[21]

Pius, in condemning artificial insemination whether by husbands or donors, had offered two principal considerations. His first objection was that insemination outside the natural act of sexual intercourse would be "to convert the domestic hearth, sanctuary of the family, into nothing more than a biological laboratory."[22] He argued that artificial insemination transforms the generating of new human life from an act of procreation into an act of reproduction and that, for this alone, it is dehumanizing and depersonalizing. It was evidently his judgment that artificial insemination drives a wedge between the unitive and procreative meanings of human sexual intercourse, sundering a union that is divinely intended to be inherent and inseparable by human agency. Obviously artificial insemination by a donor drives these two meanings of human sexual intercourse much farther apart than artificial insemination by the husband, but the difference between the two forms is only one of degree or distance.

The second reason for Pius's condemnation of artificial insemination, whether by donor or husband, was that it entails an immoral means for procuring the sperm. (This was explicitly brought forward for rejecting AIH, but obviously it applies to AID as well.)[23] In addition, Pius argued that AID violates the marital covenant and the "natural law and divine positive law," requiring that "the procreation of new life can be only the fruit of marriage."[24]

Thus *one* of the reasons why Pius XII condemned AIH was because this practice (which ought to be clearly distinguished from "assisted insemination") involves masturbation to obtain the sperm for the insemination.

Today, a number of leading Catholic moral theologians disagree with this belief. For them, AIH may be wrong on other grounds, but it is not necessarily wrong on the grounds that it involves masturbation. Most of these theologians would readily grant that an act of masturbation is involved, in the sense that the easiest way to secure the semen for fertilization is to have the husband manipulate his penis so that ejaculation occurs. · Yet they argue that this is in no sense a morally evil act; it is masturbation *in a physical sense* but is not necessarily to be considered as *morally* reprehensible.

Among Roman Catholic authors who take this position are such well-known theologians as Charles Curran,[25] John Dedek,[26] and Bernard Häring.[27] They concur in the judgment of the outstanding German Protestant ethicist, Helmut Thielicke, who wrote as follows:

> In homologous insemination . . . this objection [that the deed is wrong because it involves masturbation] is hardly valid, since it is based upon a theologically untenable doctrine of works. For Reformation thinking, at any rate, the worth or unworth of a "work" depends not upon its isolated form as such, what contemporary Roman Catholic authors would call its *physical structure,* but rather upon the state in which the person is with respect to God, and also the intention or purpose he is pursuing in this work or act. . . . Masturbation is as a rule regarded as offensive for the following reasons. First and above all because in masturbation sex is separated from the I–Thou relationship and thus loses its meaning as being the expression and consummation of this fellowship. Second, because the sexual phantasy is no longer bound to a real partnership and therefore roves about vagrantly. Third, because as a rule the absence of this bond leads to physical and psychic extravagance. The ethically decisive thing is therefore not the offensiveness of the physical function as such . . . but rather the personal situation that underlies the masturbation. . . . All acts which are centered not upon God and my neighbor but upon my own self are actualizations of sin. . . . Now it must be admitted that

the personal situation which underlies a masturbation for
the purpose of homologous insemination is fundamental-
ly and radically different. It is performed in the climate
of a real sexual fellowship and its purpose is the fulfillment of this sexual fellowship.[28]

These authors, who would seem to represent a growing consensus among Catholic and Protestant moral theologians, would
thus hold that AIH, even if it entails masturbation, can be a
morally justifiable way of fulfilling the legitimate desire of a
husband and wife to have a child of their own, provided, of
course, that their marital relationship is healthy and there is good
reason to believe that they will live together and provide a home
for a child who is indeed seen as the incarnation of their love
for one another.

This argument needs to be very seriously considered. It must
be granted that there is a vast moral difference between an act
of masturbation performed by someone in isolation, as an act of
self-indulgence or curiosity or release of tensions, and one performed by a husband who simply wants, together with the wife
he loves, to have a child of his own.

Despite the very real differences in these situations, I believe
it is essential to challenge the contemporary consensus that justifies masturbation by a husband in order to provide sperm for
artificial insemination. We must be realistic about this matter
and must remind ourselves of our existence as animal persons, as
bodied beings. To be a human being is to be an animal—to be
an animal with a difference from other animals, to be sure—but
it is still to be an animal. Our bodies are not instruments at-
tached to our selves, our persons. I am not one reality and my
body another. *I am a body, I am an animal.* My body and my
animality are, indeed, radically different in kind from the body
and animality of other animals, precisely because the former are
the body and the animality of that unique and special kind of
animal that a human being is; but I am nonetheless an animal,
and my body is an integral dimension of my self, my personhood.
It is not subpersonal, subhuman, an element of physical nature
that I can use apart from myself, now for one purpose, now for
another. I believe that the apologia advanced to justify masturba-

tion for AIH reflects a dualistic view of man that makes me a spirit dwelling in a body that I can "use" to secure "higher" values. This view sees the body and the sexual organs as infra- or subhuman, as nonpersonal "its" that confront the spiritual subject. This view, however, is erroneous for it fails to recognize the nature of our existence as human beings, as animal persons, as animals with a difference.

Nor may we forget that if a human male is to ejaculate semen, he has to do something to his body; he has to think certain thoughts and engage in various fantasies. Ejaculating sperm into a test tube is not analogous to spitting into a spittoon.

Thus a principal objection to the apologia for well-intentioned masturbation is that it implies a dualistic understanding of the human person. It repudiates, as it were, our animality and fails to consider the psychosexual dynamics in an act of masturbation.

In addition, all admit that AIH, achieved through masturbation, separates the unitive and procreative meanings of marital intercourse. We readily admit that this is done for a good purpose, to relieve the human estate and to enable persons to fulfill legitimate desires. But to justify the procedure on this ground is to accept a "proportionate good" type of ethics, according to which we can rightfully intend an evil if a proportionate or greater good can be achieved by so intending. This ethics is a variant of consequentialism and is not in accord with the type of ethics set forth in the Introduction.*

Finally, some reflections are in order about a key assumption made by ethicists who accept masturbation as a way of legitimately fulfilling the human desire of a husband and wife to have a child of their own. All agree in repudiating deeds that are malicious,[29] and they seem to locate the maliciousness of an act of masturbation in the *intent* of the agent. Finding this maliciousness of intent absent in masturbation for AIH, they conclude that the deed is in no way malicious and is therefore in no way wrong.[30]

---

*Specific objections to this "proportionate good" ethics will be developed at the conclusion of this chapter, where I will seek to show how it differs from the type of ethics outlined in the Introduction. See also chapter 6, pp. 131–158.

There is a sense, of course, in which the maliciousness that makes us sinners is rooted in the intent, in the heart. After all, Jesus tells us, "Do you not see that nothing that enters a man from outside can make him impure? It does not penetrate his being, but enters his stomach only and passes into the latrine. . . . What emerges from within a man, that and nothing else is what makes him impure" (Mk 7:18–23).

But how do we get to be malicious at heart? None of us, I believe, deliberately sets out to become a malicious person, a human being of hardened heart. What happens is that we gradually blind our eyes and stop our ears to the truth of our existence as human beings and fall into ways of acting and thinking that cripple us and, gradually, make it very difficult for us even to recognize what is wrong, and render us impotent in our struggle to do what we come to know we ought to do.

Moreover, there is an indispensable and inevitable connection between the deeds we freely choose to do and our moral identity. At times these deeds are an expression of our identity—and in this way an act of murder by a person who has already become a killer is an expression of his moral identity. At other times these deeds do not so much express an identity that we have already taken upon ourselves but, rather, start us on the path—if we freely, to some degree, choose to do them—that inevitably leads us to become what we will become. In this way, for instance, a visit to a prostitute by a man who "hates himself" for doing it can launch him on a path that will inevitably (unless he has a change of heart) lead him to take upon himself the identity of an adulterer, a person who delights in visiting prostitutes.

I believe that reflections of this kind are relevant and that theologians who have been led to justify well-intentioned masturbation by a husband (in order to provide sperm to inseminate his wife) have failed to take the relationship between act and being seriously. For the act remains an act of masturbation; it is an act, moreover, not of an angelic spirit but of an animal-person, an animal with a difference, who must think certain thoughts and manipulate his own body-person. The "justification" for this benevolent masturbation is made on the grounds of proportionate reason, but it fails to take seriously our nature as animals and it drives a wedge between the unitive and the procreative meanings of human sexual intercourse.[31]

Artificial Insemination by Donor (AID)

If AIH is to be judged wrong, then, *a fortiori,* artificial insemination by a donor, or AID, is wrong. Although this is true, it is instructive to look into this practice.

Traditionally, of course, Roman Catholic moralists condemned this practice because it involves masturbation and transforms human procreation into laboratory reproduction. Moreover, Roman Catholic and Protestant moralists have held that AID constitutes an act of adultery and hence is to be repudiated.[32] Today, however, many serious ethicists, both Protestant and Roman Catholic, question this stance. We have seen that some have found an entirely different meaning in an act of masturbation performed in isolation and one performed by a husband for the purpose of inseminating his wife, who desperately wants a child of her own, and this argument has been developed by others[33] to justify masturbation by a donor. The argument continues by claiming that adultery, in any morally significant sense, is not involved if the marital relationship is stable, the husband is willing to consent to the procedure, and it is the only (or most reasonable) way to cure the heartache and agony that a woman experiences who desperately wants to have a child of her own and cannot because her husband is infertile.[34]

It is obvious that I disagree with the reasoning of those who justify masturbation for AID. Although I believe that this practice also ruptures the marital covenant,[35] I will prescind from this question to call attention to other very relevant factors that show why AID is wrong.

AID necessarily requires the involvement of a third person, the donor, who is biologically the father of the child who is conceived as a result of the artificial insemination. Society does not, and for very good reasons, hold males in esteem who generate new human lives and then abandon them and their mothers. In AID the "donor" is *required* to do this. If he were to have concern for the child and the mother, terrible problems would ensue.

It is precisely to avoid these problems that the donor (who is quite adequately remunerated for his services) is kept anonymous. AID thus requires that the donor (even on the supposition that he is acting altruistically) be put in a position into which one *ought not* put a fellow human being: wherein he must abandon human relationships and the obligations attendant thereon that are brought into being by his free choice and activity.

It is sometimes argued that the donor is in a position analogous to that of a person who gives another a pint of blood, but the analogy is not a good one. In AID the "gift" results in the generation of a new human being, who has needs to be met and ties to the donor, and to whom the donor has ties, for the donor is in fact his father. He is a parent of the child, who is conceived as a result of the donor's free choice but for whom he will exercise no fathering at all, either prenatally or postnatally. He has communicated life to a new human being, but he has done so in a mechanistic, impersonal way and he is, in virtue of the situation in which he is placed and which he has chosen to enter, proscribed from sharing his life with the life he has brought into being by his activity. There can be no real bonds of life and love between the child and the donor, but these bonds *ought* to be real if human beings are properly to take responsibility for the foreseeable consequences of their deeds.

To ask a human being to put himself in the position of the donor, therefore, is to require him to repudiate very serious moral obligations of responsibility, love, and trust that he cannot, as a moral being, repudiate. Thus it depersonalizes and dehumanizes him. In truth, the donor's role is purely mechanistic in AID. If the sperm could be obtained by putting coins in a vending machine, surely those who are desperately anxious to have it would use this means, which shows that the donor is simply an object, a thing, a machine.

I realize that fatherhood is much more than a biological function and that many men who are not biologically the fathers of their children are truly fathers to them. But biological fatherhood is not related merely accidentally or meaninglessly to human fatherhood; the biological father has a *moral obligation* to exercise full human fatherhood toward the children he has begotten through his deeds; he has a *moral obligation* to have concern, feeling, affection, and love for the woman who, with him, has communicated life to a new human being, a new being of moral worth. AID makes these very real moral obligations mere fictions; it depersonalizes the donor, threatens the well-being of the child unnecessarily, and totally separates the unitive and procreative meanings of human sexual intercourse. These factors alone are sufficient, in my judgment, to show that AID is inherently dehumanizing and immoral, prescinding entirely from the serious questions of masturbation by the donor and infidelity on the part of the wife.

At times, because of very tragic conditions, the biological father and/or mother of a child may be forced to offer their child for adoption, but this is quite different from AID. In the tragic instances when a man or woman has begotten a child whom he or she must give up for adoption, the factors that lead them to contemplate this step are profoundly different from those that face the donor in AID. In AID a human freely chooses to initiate an act that he foresees will result in the conception and birth of a child—who is indeed his and to whom he is really, not fictitiously, related, and for whom he is to have no human, fatherly concern. This need not be true in adoption.[36]

It is pertinent to note that this practice ruptures the covenant between husband and wife. When a man and a woman marry they give themselves to one another and receive one another unconditionally. They give themselves to one another so completely that they are no longer two but one; they are summoned to a communion in being. They are called upon to love one another with a love that is willing to accept burdens, to be self-sacrificial when the times require, and to be willing to forego the fulfillment of legitimate desires if such achievement would require them to repudiate the personhood of the other. AID tears the fabric of the marital covenant, for it is a rejection of the husband, objectively, even if this is not subjectively recognized in conscious awareness.

The husband, through no fault of his own, but simply by being the person he is and the one whom his wife accepted and to whom she committed herself, is incapable of helping her have the child that he and she desire. The donor cannot help her have *this* child, for the child whom she and her husband desire (or ought to desire) is the image of their love for one another, flesh of their flesh, bone of their bone. AID implies rejection of the personhood of the husband and establishes conditions that *can* (even if they actually *may* not) threaten the stability of the marriage and the well-being of the child. These risks are deliberately brought into existence as a result of human choices, made to fulfill the woman's desire to bear a child of her own, even if this means exercising parenthood with someone other than her husband, with someone who will never care for her or for the child.

Test-Tube Fertilization, Cloning, and Other "Reproductive" Technologies

It is obvious that the *human* significance of sexual intercourse as an act that is expressive of the love between husband and wife (its unitive dimension) and inherently capable of generating new human life (its procreative meaning) is repudiated by test-tube or *in vitro* fertilization, embryo banks, surrogate mothers, cloning, and other reproductive techniques. All of these practices sever the inherently intelligible relationship between the unitive and procreative meanings of sexual union. But even if we prescind from this very significant moral fact, other considerations show why these practices are inherently immoral and, consequently, ought never be adopted, unless one is also willing to adopt a consequentialist mentality, either quantitative or qualitative, in ethics.[37] We can set forth these considerations by dealing in depth with test-tube fertilization.

Ramsey has argued, and in my judgment correctly, that the "making" of babies through this method is inherently evil inasmuch as it is unjust experimentation on a future, possible child. Even if we omit the consideration of abortion (for test-tube fertilization and cloning demand the abortion of "abnormal" embryos deliberately brought into existence through these procedures), we must conclude that test-tube fertilization cannot exclude damage to the child-to-be, to the child who is to be brought into existence through this procedure. We cannot even come to know, Ramsey insists, whether damage will be done by the manipulation of ova, fertilized ova, and developing embryos unless we are *willing to inflict damage* in order to find out.[38]

Test-tube fertilization is clearly *not* therapeutic. It is a purely experimental, research procedure, of no possible medical benefit to the "subject," that is, the child-to-be. No disease is diagnosed or cured or prevented as a result of the procedure; there is really no "patient."

Two leading advocates of test-tube fertilization, Paul Edwards and Robert Steptoe, argue that the woman who wants a child of her own and is incapable of having one through coital intercourse is the "patient" and that the procedure is intended to cure her "disease." But they are simply abusing language in making this argument. The woman in question is not a patient in any meaningful sense of that term. The experiments *in vitro* are not exercised on *her;* they expose *her* to no risks (although possibly the laparoscopy, whereby an ovum is removed from her ovaries, does this). On the contrary, these experiments are done to a living being who is brought into existence by fertilizing her ovum. The "patient," in other words, is a developing human being, a child-to-be, and this being does *not* suffer from any malady that could be cured by the experiments.

In fact, the very effort to bring this child into existence entails the risk that he will be harmed, perhaps irreparably, and this risk cannot be excluded. Test-tube fertilization can be carried out *only* if the experimenters are *willing* to inflict damage on the child-to-be, damage that may not be observed until years later. As a result, Ramsey writes, "*in vitro* fertilization constitutes unethical medical experimentation on possible future human beings, and therefore . . . is subject to absolute moral prohibition."[39]

Test-tube fertilization cannot exclude the possibility of severely damaging the child-to-be. But "unless the *possibility* of such damage can be definitively excluded," Ramsey continues, "*in vitro* fertilization is an immoral experiment on possible future human beings . . . [and] this condition cannot be met, at least not by the first 'successful' cases; and therefore . . . any man's or any woman's venture to begin human life in this way is morally forbidden. We cannot morally *get to know* how to perfect this technique to relieve human infertility."[40] Researchers cannot "*exclude* the possibility that they will do irreparable damage to the child to be."[41] They cannot know, or ever come to know, what they are doing to a possible future child. Since they cannot have this knowledge without treating this possible future human being as a purely experimental animal (which a future human child, a being of moral worth, definitely is *not*), the very effort to gain this knowledge is immoral since it demands that the experimenters be willing to inflict damage on a future possible child in order to find out whether their experiments will in fact do so.

In addition, as Leon Kass perceptively notes, test-tube fertilization is not the only alternative to alleviating infertility in women because of a pathological disorder that affects the Fallopian tubes. It is possible in a number of cases to reconstruct the Fallopian tubes surgically, as has been done successfully in 30 percent of such cases.[42] This alternative to test-tube fertilization is truly therapeutic, is not purely experimental, and does not sever the procreative from the unitive dimension of human sexual intercourse.[43]

It is not to our purpose to discuss cloning or the other reproductive technologies that are being advocated. All are like test-tube fertilization in that they constitute unjustifiable experimentations on a possible future child. All sever the relationship between the unitive and procreative meanings of human sexual intercourse—indeed, sever it in such a way that the generation of human life becomes a manufacturing process, a matter of "reproduction." It is inherently meaningful that the generation of new human beings is *not* a matter of manufacturing or reproducing but of procreating. As procreation, the generation of new human life is understood, and properly, not as an activity that results in a "product" but as an activity whereby a man and a woman who share their life and love through sexual intercourse at the very same time and in the very same act communicate and share life and love with a future human generation.

Human beings, created words of the living and loving God who sent us his Son, his Uncreated Word, to be one with us and for us, are, like the Uncreated Word in whose image they are created, to be begotten, not made, and they are to be begotten by a man and a woman whose abiding love for one another reaches out to the future and will provide the room where new human life can grow and be given the conditions under which it will flourish and achieve its fullness.

The position developed within this chapter has been eloquently stated by Leon Kass in a very perceptive essay that is concerned with the "new beginnings of life" and the desire to relieve the human estate by adopting the technologies for generating life in the laboratory.

> The price to be paid for the "optimum" baby is the transfer of procreation from the home to the laboratory and its coincident transformation into manufacture. Increasing control over the product is purchased by the increasing depersonalization of the process. The complete depersonalization of procreation shall be, in itself, seriously dehumanizing no matter how optimum the product. It should not be forgotten that human procreation not only issues human beings, but is itself a human activity.[44]

Those who share Robert Francoeur's enthusiasm for the "technological imperative"[45] and Joseph Fletcher's belief that the more rationally controlled a process, the more human it is,[46] will find our position "antediluvian," the querulous and worrisome fruit of a "mystical" or "metaphysical" frame of mind.[47] But those who share the conviction that what our actions tell us about ourselves is far more important than what they bring about in the way of consequences will recognize that our position is by no means nostalgic sentimentality or a repudiation of human technology but is rooted in an understanding of the human person as a being who is an animal of a special kind, a living image of God. As animals, we are able to "reproduce" our kind, but as animals with a difference, by reason of being images of the living and loving God, we are to communicate life and love to a future generation through acts of loving procreation, through engendering deeds that communicate God's covenant of life and love to the generating generations of mankind.

Some Roman Catholic authors[48] may also be disappointed with the conclusions reached in this chapter. They reject the utilitarian ethics advocated by Fletcher but they believe that, at times, for the sake of very important human values, some of the procedures discussed in this chapter can be justified even if they require the direct intention of some measure of evil. Thus it seems necessary to conclude with a note on the ethics of the proportionate good, since it is so pervasive today.

The Ethics of the Proportionate Good

We have noted that this ethics has been given its clearest articulation by Richard McCormick, who discerns it in the writings of William Van der Marck, Cornelius Van der Poel, Bruno Schüller, Louis Janssens, and others.[49] It is also reflected in the work of John Dedek[50] and, to some extent, that of Bernard Häring.[51] Although Charles Curran is not a member of this school of thought, he has sympathies with it, and a number of his positions on bioethical questions could be supported by this ethical position.[52]

According to this view, it is morally permissible directly to intend a "non-moral" (or "pre-moral" or "ontic") evil, such as death or the sterilization of a person or his wounding, so long as there is a "proportionate" reason for doing so. As McCormick expresses it, "Where a higher good is at stake and the only means to protect it is to choose to do a nonmoral evil, then the will remains properly disposed to the values constitutive of the human good. . . . This is to say that the intentionality is good even when the person, reluctantly and regretfully to be sure, intends the nonmoral evil if a truly proportionate reason for such a choice is present."[53]

Putting it another way, McCormick maintains that one can justly do a deed by which a human good is destroyed in a human being, and by which this destruction is directly intended by the doer, so long as there is a proportionate reason. He writes:

> Would it not be clearer and more precise to say that it is legitimate to intend premoral evil *in ordine—ad finem proportionatum?* I may choose and intend the pain of a child or a patient if it is the only way or the most reasonable way to secure his greater good. This "greater good" does not mean that the premoral disvalue is not intended; it means that it is not intended *propter se.* Therefore, would it not be better to say that it is legitimate to intend a disvalue *in se sed non propter se?* When

there is no proportionate reason, the disvalue caused is
chosen and intended *in se et propter se* and it is this
propter se which makes the act immoral.[54]

Appealing to the ethics of the proportionate good, several
authors have tentatively justified both AIH and AID and test-
tube fertilization,[55] and it is evident that this type of ethics can
be used to justify such procedures. According to the ethics of
the proportionate good, the only *inherently* evil acts are those
that are formally defined as such, for instance, blaspheming God,
causing another to sin (causing *moral* evil, as opposed to pre-moral
evil), murder (= unjust,—i.e., disproportionate—killing), etc.[56]

This type of ethics, in my judgment, ought to be rejected. It
is, as McCormick admits, a type of consequentialism. It fails to
take seriously the inner or inherent intelligibility of our acts and
can be criticized on many grounds.

First, it seems that even utilitarian consequentialists (such as
Fletcher) would agree that one ought not to intend an evil such
as death in itself and for itself. No one, however, really intends
an evil in and for itself; one always intends his act to result in
the participation of some real good. Even a person who cruelly
tortures another, because this is an exquisitely delightful experience for the former, does not intend the torture in and for itself.
Although his will is directly targeted on the torture, he intends
the torture for the esthetic experience it will bring him.

Second, if we take seriously the significance of our deeds as
revelations of our being and as shaping our moral identity, we
must conclude that if our will is targeted directly on an evil, such
as death, we must be willing to take on, as part of our moral
identity, the identity of a killer, even if this is only reluctantly
and regretfully accepted. We take on the identity of evildoers as
part of our identity, for this is what we *do* if the evil cannot not
be intended.

Third, if we look upon the significance of our deeds from a
Christian perspective, mindful of being living images of God, we
realize that we ought to be true images of him. God, who is absolutely innocent of evil, *permits* evil but does not directly intend
it (McCormick explicitly acknowledges the real difference between an intending and a permitting will).[57] If we are to be a

faithful image of God, then we, too, should not choose to do a deed that of necessity requires us to intend the evil that is effected, for if we do, we cannot be absolutely innocent of evil.

The ethics of proportionate good, as noted, is a type of consequentialism. This means that it is more interested in what our actions get done (their "consequences") than in what they tell us about ourselves. The formula advocated by McCormick, namely, that we may rightfully intend evil in itself for the sake of attaining a proportionate end (*in se in ordine ad finem proportionatum*),[58] is another way of saying that the end justifies the means.

According to this ethics, human acts (aside from those that can be designated wicked in a formal sense) are neither inherently good nor inherently wicked. Rape, for example, is a wicked act only because there is no proportionate good to justify it; but, in theory, rape could be justifiable in the presence of a proportionate good.[59] This means that human acts become good or evil by reason of something other than themselves: the presence or absence of a due good. This position is very contradictory to the position set forth in the Introduction.

There are, unfortunately, times when we bring about evil no matter what we do or do not do. We can, as Christians and as human beings, do a deed that causes evil if there is a proportionate reason for doing so, but in such instances our intent must be on the good that is achievable in and through the deed. The evil is only an unavoidable concomitant of the act that is targeted on the good. It is not possible to go more fully into this very important matter here; however, I believe that the difference between the ethics of proportionate good and the ethics advocated throughout this study, which is concerned with the inherent intelligibility of our acts as revelatory of our being, ought to be clear to the reader. For fuller analyses of the issues the reader is urged to consult the literature cited in the following footnote,[60] as well as the reflections in chapter 6.

Chapter 2

1. See Lawrence Fuchs, *Family Matters* (New York: Random House, 1972), chap. 1.

2. On this see George Gilder, *Sexual Suicide* (New York: Quadrangle, 1973).

3. On this see Paul F. Palmer, "Christian Marriage: Contract or Covenant?" *Theological Studies,* 33 (December 1972):617–665. See also Paul Ramsey, "On Taking Sexual Responsibility Seriously Enough," in his *Deeds and Rules in Christian Ethics* (New York: Scribner's, 1967), pp. 11f.

4. Paul Ramsey, *Fabricated Man* (New Haven: Yale University Press, 1970), pp. 32–34.

5. See "Documentation Syntheticum de Moralitate Regulationis Nativitatum," popularly called the "majority report" of the Pontifical Commission on Population, Family, and Births. It is printed ·in Robert Hoyt, ed., *The Birth Control Debate* (Kansas City, Mo.: National Catholic Reporter, 1969), pp. 79–101.

6. Fletcher's thoughts on the relationship between "baby making" and "love making," which he terms the procreative (or rather, "reproductive") and the unitive dimensions of human sexual intercourse, are set forth in many places. Note in particular his essay "Ethical Aspects of Genetic Controls," *New England Journal of Medicine,* 285 (1971):776–783, and his *The Ethics of Genetic Control: Ending Reproductive Roulette* (New York: Doubleday Anchor, 1974).

7. The Francoeur's views are found in several recent works, among them *Hot Sex: Cool Sex* (New York: Harcourt Brace Jovanovich, 1975).

8. Ashley Montagu, *Sex, Culture, and Man* (New York: Knopf, 1972), in particular chap. 1.

9. Gilder, *op. cit.,* pp. 32–34.

10. Leon Kass, *Making Babies—The New Biology and the "Old" Morality* (Hastings-on-Hudson, N.Y.: Institute of Society, Ethics and the Life Sciences, 1972), no pagination. This originally appeared as an essay in the winter 1972 issue of *Public Interest* and was reprinted, with additions and modifications, in *Genetics and the Future of Man,* Michael Hamilton, ed. (Grand Rapids: Eerdmans, 1972). See also Leon Kass, "The New Biology: What Price Relieving the Human Estate?" *Science,* vol. 174 (Nov. 19, 1971).

11. Gerald Leach, *The Biocrats* (Baltimore: Pelican, 1972), pp. 80–117.

12. Gordon Rattray Taylor, *The Biological Time-bomb* (Cleveland: World, 1968).

13. Albert Rosenfeld, *The Second Genesis* (Englewood Cliffs, N.J.: Prentice-Hall, 1968).

14. See, e.g., *Time* cover story, "The New Genetics: Man Into Superman (Apr. 19, 1971).

15. See R. G. Edwards, "Aspects of Human Reproduction," in Watson Fuller, ed., *The Biological Revolution: Social Good or Social Evil?* (New York: Doubleday Anchor, 1971), pp. 130ff.

16. Leach, *op. cit.,* p. 82.

17. *Ibid.,* p. 85.

18. *Ibid.,* p. 82.

19. Pius XII, "Address to the Fourth International Convention of Catholic Doctors," Sept. 29, 1949, *Acta Apostolicae Sedis,* 41 (1949): 559–560. On this matter see Gerald Kelly S.J., *Medico-Moral Problems* (St. Louis: Catholic Hospital Association, 1957), pp. 239–244. Kelly gives the text of Pius's address on pp. 228–230.

20. Kelly, *op. cit.*

21. *Ibid.*

22. Pius XII, "Address to the Congress of the Italian Catholic Union of Midwives," Nov. 26, 1951, *Acta Apostolicae Sedis,* 43 (1951):850. Cited in Kelly, *op. cit.,* p. 230. On these papal declarations see also John F. Dedek, *Contemporary Medical Ethics* (New York: Sheed and Ward, 1975), pp. 97–100.

23. Pius XII, "Address to the Fourth International Convention of Catholic Doctors," *loc. cit.,* in Kelly, *op. cit.,* p. 229.

24. *Ibid.*

25. Charles E. Curran, *Politics, Medicine, and Christian Ethics: A Dialogue with Paul Ramsey* (Philadelphia: Fortress Press, 1973), pp. 192–194, 213ff. Curran's position is developed on pp. 217–218.

26. John Dedek, *op. cit.,* pp. 92–102. Dedek offers a good survey of contemporary developments in Roman Catholic moral theology concerning AIH, citing the views of Rodger Van Allen, Richard McCormick, and others. His own conclusion seems to state the consensus adequately: "I . . . think that AIH generally should be excluded unless it is the only way an otherwise sterile couple can achieve procreation. If in particular cases it is required for procreation, masturbation would seem to be a morally acceptable technique of obtaining sperm from the husband, since the moral meaning of the physical act is derived from the circumstances and purpose toward which it is directed" (p. 101).
Although I agree that intentionality and other circumstances can change the moral species of the same outward act (e.g., intercourse as an act expressing the love of husband and wife or intercourse as the exploitation of a young girl), it is necessary to distinguish clearly

between an agent's *intent* and his *motive*. In AIH the *motive* is certainly good (to help one's wife have a child that both husband and wife ardently desire), but the *intent*, both of the agent and the act (*finis operis*), is to masturbate, and this remains the relevant moral species of the act in question.

27. Bernard Häring. *Medical Ethics* (South Bend: Fides, 1972), p. 91f.

28. Helmut Thielicke, *The Ethics of Sex* (New York: Harper & Row, 1964), pp. 255–256.

29. See discussions in the authors cited in notes 25–27.

30. Here it is very instructive to consult Curran, *op. cit.*, pp. 200–219.

31. Criticism of the type of moral methodology operative in Curran, Dedek, Häring, and other contemporary Roman Catholic moral theologians is more fully articulated in my article, "Sex, Love, and Procreation," *Homiletic and Pastoral Review* (May 1976). Reprinted in the *Synthesis Series* by Franciscan Herald Press.

32. See, e.g., Kelly, *op. cit.*, pp. 231–239.

33. See, e.g., Curran, *op. cit.*, pp. 217f.

34. Here it useful to consult an advocate of this practice, James Nelson, in his *Human Medicine* (Minneapolis: Augsburg, 1975).

35. See below, p. 00.

36. On this entire subject it is very useful to consult Ramsey, *Fabricated Man*, pp. 130–138; Kelly, *op. cit.*, pp. 231–239; Thielicke, *op. cit.*, pp. 258–268.

37. Obviously, those who adopt a consequentialist position will be willing, if certain kinds of goods are achievable by test-tube fertilization, to justify this procedure. They may say that as a general practice it is immoral, that there may, in the concrete, be no good basis for justifying it, but they have already justified the practice *in principle* because, in principle, every kind of deed is theoretically justifiable on a consequentialist model.

38. Ramsey, "Shall We 'Reproduce'?" *Journal of the American Medical Association*, 220 (June 5, 1972):1346.

39. *Ibid.*, p. 1347.

40. *Ibid.*

41. *Ibid.*

42. Leon Kass, "New Beginnings of Life," in Hamilton, ed., *op. cit.*, p. 26.

43. Curran, *op. cit.,* pp. 200–219 (in particular pp. 210–219), offers a critique of the position defended by Ramsey and accepted here. Curran, while in many ways sympathetic with Ramsey, holds that at times the real good of children for a couple (the *bonum prolis*), along with the fact that risks for the well-being of a child-to-be are present in normal coitus and in the role of creativity in human life, can in very limited cases justify not only AID but test-tube fertilization. It should be pointed out that the normal risks for the child-to-be in coital intercourse are not *deliberately* brought into being by the agents, as in laboratory reproduction.

44. Kass, "The New Biology: What Price Relieving the Human Estate?" p. 784. See also Willard Gaylin, "The Frankenstein Myth Become a Reality," *New York Times Magazine,* March 5, 1972, p. 48.

45. See Robert Francoeur, "We Can—We Must: Reflections on the Technological Imperative," *Theological Studies,* 33 (September 1972): 428-439.

46. See Fletcher, "Ethical Aspects of Genetic Control," pp. 781–782.

47. This is the way Fletcher characterizes the positions of Ramsey and Kass in his *The Ethics of Genetic Control*; see pp. 30, 34, 88, 99.

48. E.g., John Dedek, Charles Curran, Bernard Häring, Richard McCormick.

49. See Richard McCormick, *Ambiguity in Moral Choice* (Marquette University Pere Marquette Lecture in Theology, 1973). McCormick names Van der Marck, Van der Poel, and Schüller as authors whose thought emerges in the ethics of the proportionate good. In his subsequent "Notes on Moral Theology" for *Theological Studies* 36 (March 1975), McCormick comments on recent work by Louis Janssens that, in his judgment, leads to the same type of ethical position.

50. Cf. the work cited in n. 22. See also Dedek's *Human Life* (New York: Sheed and Ward, 1972), chap. 1.

51. See Häring's *Medical Ethics* (South Bend: Fides, 1972) and his *Ethics of Manipulation* (New York: Seabury, 1975).

52. Charles Curran's position is somewhat complicated by his "theology of compromise," and he implies that there are inherently evil acts if acts are properly described (see his *Catholic Moral Theology in Dialogue* [South Bend: Fides, 1971], pp. 81–92). Nonetheless, he states that the type of ethics reflected in McCormick's writings and in authors who can be grouped with McCormick is congenial to his own and that he shares their viewpoint on many important issues. For this see his essay on the principle of double effect in his *Ongoing Revision* (South Bend: Fides, 1975), especially pp. 206–207. In addition, he tentatively accepts AID in some situations and even envisages

the moral use of test-tube fertilization. On this see his *Politics, Medicine, and Ethics,* pp. 200–219.

53. McCormick, *Ambiguity in Moral Choice,* p. 45.

54. McCormick, "Notes on Moral Theology," *Theological Studies,* 33 (March 1972):74–75.

55. See Dedek, *Contemporary Medical Ethics,* pp. 92–102; Curran, *Politics, Medicine, and Ethics,* pp. 200–219.

56. See McCormick, *Ambiguity in Moral Choice,* pp. 53–65.

57. *Ibid.,* pp. 57–65, 70–72.

58. See text cited in n. 54.

59. It is quite instructive to read what Daniel Maguire says about rape in his *Death by Choice* (New York: Doubleday, 1973), p. 99. Maguire appeals to McCormick's ethics of proportionate good in developing his thought, and what he says about rape is quite correct in terms of this ethics.

60. On this see Paul Ramsey, *War and the Christian Conscience* (Durham: Duke University Press, 1962), pp. 39–59; *idem,* "Abortion: A Review Article," *The Thomist,* 37 (January 1973): pp. 175–224; Germain Grisez, "Toward a Consistent Natural-Law Ethics of Killing," *American Journal of Jurisprudence,* vol. 15 (1970); *idem, Abortion: The Myths, the Realities, and the Arguments,* (New York: Corpus, 1970), chap. 6; and my *Becoming Human* (Dayton: Pflaum, 1975), chap. 4, and "Ethics and Human Identity: The Challenge of the New Biology," *Horizons: The Journal of the College Theology Society,* 3 (Spring 1976):17–37. See also my "Sterilization; Catholic Teaching and Catholic Practice," *Homiletic and Pastoral Review* (August-September, 1977).

3: Protecting the Human Genetic Pool (1): Sterilization and Contraception

The great advances in medical technology have, paradoxically, contributed to the creation of a very serious problem. Individuals who suffer from seriously crippling hereditary disorders are now able to survive childhood, marry, and have children of their own; as a result, the proportion of persons who suffer from these hereditary disorders has increased. Even more seriously, the proportion of persons who are "normal," in the sense that they do not suffer from a genetically caused disorder yet are carriers of recessive genetic disorders that can seriously cripple their children, has increased more significantly. Because of this, several research geneticists fear that the human genetic pool is deteriorating and that this deterioration will accelerate in generations to come unless measures are taken to reach a new equilibrium and reverse the direction.

This concern over the future of the human genetic pool is found in the writings of several eminent geneticists, among them the late Herman Muller, a Nobel laureate biologist from Indiana University, who feared a genetic apocalypse. He once wrote that

> it is probably true that some 20 percent, if not more, of a human population has received a genetic impairment that arose by mutation in the immediately previous generation, in addition to the far larger number of impairments inherited from earlier generations. If this is true, then, to avoid genetic deterioration about 20 percent of the population who are more heavily laden with genetic

> defects than the average must in each generation fail to live to maturity or, if they do live must fail to reproduce. Otherwise the load of genetic defects carried by that population would inevitably rise.[1]

To illustrate the problem, we can take diabetes and pyloric stenosis (two disorders that are correctable by treatment) as examples. Prior to the discovery of insulin by Banting and Best in the 1920s, a child or adolescent who developed diabetes would soon die. Now, a diabetic child or adolescent can live a long life, marry, and have children. Because of this, many experts believe that in subsequent generations insulin injection may become as common as taking aspirin or wearing glasses. Similarly, many children died of starvation in early infancy because of pyloric stenosis, a genetically caused disorder in which the muscle that closes the opening between the stomach and the small intestine is too powerful, so that when it contracts the victim vomits in projectile fashion. If untreated, the infant who suffers from this malady will soon die. But a simple surgical operation, introduced in the 1930s, snips the muscle and weakens it, effecting a permanent cure. Still, the cause of the disability is latent in the genes of the afflicted person, so that when these children mature and have children of their own, the incidence of this disability inevitably increases. The same can be said of many other disorders, among them impairments far more crippling and less amenable to surgical or chemical treatment than pyloric stenosis or diabetes, such as Duchesne muscular distrophy, cystic fibrosis, and sickle-cell anemia.

However, pessimism over the genetic future of the human race, as reflected in the writings of Muller and others, is not universally shared by the scientific community. Many agree with H. Harris, Galton Professor of Human Genetics at Cambridge University (England), that the vision of a genetic apocalypse "is often based on a somewhat naive and very simplistic idea of the mode of operation of natural selection and on an underestimation of the genetic complexity of human populations."[2] With him, they maintain that it is not proper to infer "that present advances in our understanding and treatment of inherited disorders require this grave prognostication of doom."[3] As Harris and others note, many diseases that are associated with hereditary defects, for instance, diabetes, also depend on environmental causes, so that it is possible to prevent their manifestation by environmental controls. In addition, many recessive defects differ markedly in incidence from one racial or social group to another. For example, Tay-Sachs disease occurs most frequently among Jews whose ancestors came from an area near the Baltic Sea and sickle-cell anemia among Negroes whose ancestors came from a region near Lake Victoria in Africa. As marriage between these and other groups increases, the incidence of Tay-Sachs disease and sickle-cell anemia will necessarily decrease. As Harris notes, the quality of human life may depend more on environmental and ecological factors than on hereditarily transmitted recessive defects.[4]

The position advanced by Harris and scientists of similar views seems to have much more scientific evidence in its support than the extremely gloomy position of Muller and his supporters. Nonetheless, it must be recognized that the hereditary transmission of crippling disorders poses serious moral questions, simply because knowledge increases moral responsibility. In earlier ages we did not have the knowledge we have today about the transmission of genetically induced disorders. We now know, to some extent, the hereditary basis of specific diseases (e.g., phenylketonuria, Huntington's chorea, cystic fibrosis, etc.) and the statistics that govern their incidence in the children born to couples who are carriers of the defective genes that trigger these diseases.

I am not too concerned about the transmission of hereditary maladies caused by *dominant* genes (e.g., dwarfism, retinal aplasia, epiloia), because the person who has a dominant genetic defect, as Gerald Leach observes, "knows that he has it; he knows what suffering, or otherwise, it causes him; unless he is mentally subnormal he can understand the clear risks for his children. There will be a fifty-fifty chance that they will have it."[5] I am chiefly concerned with the transmission of crippling disorders caused by *recessive* genes, and there are good reasons why concern is justified. This also applies to crippling disorders that are not strictly hereditary but are linked to chromosomal disorders or sexual identity (e.g. Down's syndrome, Turner's syndrome, Hunter's disease, etc.).

We ought to be concerned with transmission of serious disorders by "normal" parents who carry recessive genes or chromosomal defects because (1) we know that the number of persons afflicted by disabilities caused by recessive genetic defects is increasing within the general population and (2) we know, in some measure, how this is occurring. We know, as W. French Anderson of the National Institutes of Health has noted, that "15 out of every 100 newborn infants have hereditary disorders of greater or lesser severity"[6] and, as Joshua Lederberg has written, that "25 percent of our hospital beds and the places in our institutions are occupied by persons suffering some degree of genetic disease."[7] We cannot hide from these statistics or from the fact that a specifiable number of children, born of couples with recessive genes or chromosomal abnormalities, will be handicapped, at times quite seriously, by a disability caused by those genes or chromosomes. Thus we must seek to determine what can be done to remedy the situation.

Positive Eugenics

Some writers (notably Muller and Lederberg) who take a dismal view of the genetic future of mankind are in favor of an aggressive policy of "positive" eugenics. They believe that an all-out effort could improve the human genetic pool and they advocate such measures as artificial insemination by donor (Muller), test-tube fertilization, sperm and/or ovum banks, and the cloning of individuals of outstanding traits (Lederberg) as means to achieve this goal.

We have already considered some of the moral issues raised by these technologies and have argued that they are dehumanizing insofar as they transform a human activity, procreation, into a laboratory technique, reproduction. We also argued that they necessarily involve unethical experimentation on children-to-be, requiring the abortion of fetuses that are deliberately brought into existence and crippled by the decision to use these technologies, which sunder the inherent relationship between the unitive and procreative meanings of human sexual intercourse. In addition, the attempts of positive eugenics to cope with the problem of the genetic future of mankind are not, in the judgment of many competent scientists, realistic. That is, hopes of protecting the human genetic pool by "breeding in" good traits are not well grounded scientifically. As Leach put it:

> Few biologists would go to the stake asserting, for instance, that the Bach family was thick with musical genes or that Gandhi inherited his value system at conception. . . . Breeding for all-round improvement is out. . . . There are simply too many biological arguments against it.[8]

Leach says that selective breeding for *specific* characteristics is possible to some extent, inasmuch as "there are several important qualities where genes do at least set the upper and lower limits of the potential on which environment and upbringing can work."[9] Nevertheless, it would appear that positive, aggressive efforts to "breed in" good qualities would be a misdirection of human energy. As Hudson Hoagland, a noted biologist, has written, "We know too little about the human genotype to feel confidence in our ability to do anything to modify it in favor of desirable traits."[10]

The same point is illustrated in a homely way by a story (undoubtedly apocryphal) related of Bernard Shaw, when he was approached by a dancer who suggested that they "make babies" since the infants would have her beautiful body and Shaw's magnificent mind. Shaw, it is related, responded by saying, "Yes, but what if they had *my* body and *your* brains?"

Positive eugenics, therefore, does not seem to be a proper means, morally or pragmatically, to solve the critical problems concerning the quality of future human life. *Negative* or *therapeutic* (or at least *preventive*) eugenics, however, offers more realistic and, as shall become clearer as we proceed, more humane ways of coping with these problems. The purpose of "negative" eugenics is to prevent, if possible, the transmission of genetically induced disorders to a future human generation. But even in negative or preventive eugenics there are very serious moral questions, and not all of the methods are morally justifiable.

Forms of negative eugenics have been proposed that demand critical attention, and we shall be occupied with the more prominent of these means in this and the following chapters. We shall consider (1) eugenic sterilization and contraception, (2) "screening" fetal populations and aborting fetuses discovered to be suffering from genetically induced disorders, and (3) genetic therapy or gene surgery, genetic counseling, and responsible parenthood. I am not attempting, in proposing these forms of negative eugenics, to exhaust all the proposals that have been or can be made, nor does it follow that these proposals are mutually exclusive. For instance, genetic counseling is often coupled with amniocentesis and "therapeutic" abortion. Because the listing is a conspectus of proposals that loom large in the literature and practice of negative eugenics, these proposals form the basis for our discussion and we turn first to eugenic sterilization and contraception.

Eugenic Sterilization and Contraception

Traditionally, Roman Catholic moral theologians held that sterilization is morally permissible only when it is "indirect," that is, when the sterilizing effect of an act is not its direct purpose or the intent of the agent. They thus permitted sterilization when "the excision of a generative organ for a diseased condition which threatens the life or physical welfare of a patient" was necessary and when there was a "medically sound reason for the operation."[11] As John Dedek has noted, however, when the traditional argument against direct sterilization was analyzed "the real reason for opposition to the act was disclosed." This "real reason" was that sterilization—aside from instances when the generative organs were diseased or threatened by a disease such as cancer—is contraceptive, interfering with "the procreative purpose of sexual intercourse."[12] In other words, direct sterilization was traditionally proscribed by Roman Catholic moral theologians because it is contraceptive, and contraception was regarded as inherently immoral. For this reason it is proper to consider the moral issues raised by eugenic sterilization and contraception together.[13]

Although the Roman Catholic Church still teaches authoritatively that contraception and direct sterilization are inherently immoral,[14] it must be acknowledged that several prominent Roman Catholic moral theologians, with the great majority of Protestant theologians, justify contraception and direct sterilization for eugenic purposes.[15] Indeed, the justification advanced by some Roman Catholic writers for direct eugenic sterilization is predicated upon the same kind of moral analysis by which they have justified contraception. It is thus necessary to examine this question very carefully, and we can begin by looking at an argument advanced by the noted German Catholic moral theologian, Bernard Häring, to justify direct sterilization for eugenic purposes, that is, to prevent conception of a child who might be seriously handicapped by a disorder caused by the recessive genes of his parents. Häring writes as follows:

> Traditional moral theology has consistently distinguished between direct and indirect sterilization. Any sterilization with the stated intention of inducing a temporary or irreversible sterility was declared immoral, while sterilization necessary for healing organic ailments was declared licit. This approach, though sensible, is too narrow. The vocabulary is hardly intelligible to medical thought today in view of the fact that the Church has given official sanction and encouragement to the principle of responsible parenthood, and has realized the tremendous relevance of marital relationships to the stability of a marriage and to the health and harmonious relationship of husband and wife. It might be said, then, that the real immorality comes in the irresponsible refusal to fulfill the vocation of husband and wife and of mother and father. The intention to carry out this base decision by sterilization must be absolutely rejected. But wherever the direct preoccupation is responsible care for the health of persons or for saving a marriage (which also affects the total health of all persons involved), sterilization can then receive its justification from valid medical reasons. If therefore a competent physician can determine, in full agreement with his patient, that in this particular situation a new pregnancy must be excluded now and forever because it would be thoroughly irresponsible, and if from a medical point of view sterilization is the best possible solution, it cannot be against the principles of medical ethics, nor is it against "natural law". . . . The medical decision, however, cannot disregard the foreseeable or possible effects of vasectomy or tubal ligation upon the total health of the person subjected to the procedure.[16]

Although Häring, in this passage, does not explicitly relate sterilization for eugenic purposes to contraception, he justifies direct sterilization for the same moral reasons that have been advanced by numerous writers, both Catholic and Protestant (including Häring himself),[17] to justify contraception under certain conditions. In fact, such contemporary Catholic moral theologians as Charles Curran[18] and John Dedek[19] justify voluntary eugenic sterilization because they have concluded that contraceptive intercourse, under certain conditions, is morally justifiable. They note that the chief difference between a contraceptive such as the pill and a sterilizing operation such as a vasectomy or tubal ligation is that the former is temporary and reversible whereas the latter is more permanent, usually irreversible, and can have psychological effects on individuals that do not occur in the use of other contraceptives.[20] (Here it ought to be noted that a new type of sterilization for women has been developed recently, the so-called rubber-band procedure, which is easily reversible.)

Indeed, it could be said that most Protestant and many Catholic authors agree that voluntary eugenic sterilization is morally justifiable if this is the best *medical* way of preventing the conception of children who are likely to be afflicted with serious disorders caused by the recessive genes of their parents—and this agreement ensues precisely because these authors agree that contraception can be justified for good reasons.[21] It can also be said, I believe, that the population at large, including most Catholics, holds that contraception is not inherently evil and can be practiced if there are good reasons for doing so.

Yet this consensus, on the popular level and among reputable moral theologians both Protestant and Catholic, does not settle the matter. It is imperative to examine the question of contraception and voluntary eugenic sterilization and to look critically at the arguments advanced in their support. First, however, we will look at the relevant sections of the encyclical *Humanae Vitae,* in which Pope Paul VI reaffirmed the traditional teaching of the Church that contraception is inherently evil.

> These acts, by which husband and wife are united in
> chaste intimacy and by means of which human life is
> transmitted, are, as the Council recalled, "noble and

worthy," and they do not cease to be lawful if, *for causes independent of the will of husband and wife,* they are foreseen to be infecund, since they always remain ordered toward expressing and consolidating their union. In fact, as experience bears witness, not every conjugal act is followed by a new life. God has wisely disposed natural laws and rhythms of fecundity which, of themselves, cause a separation in the succession of births. Nonetheless, the Church, calling men back to the observance of the natural law, as interpreted by their constant doctrine, teaches that *each and every marriage act must remain open to the transmission of life.*[22]

It should be noted that the Pope recognizes that an act of marital intercourse is good even if there is no procreative intent and even if procreation is impossible. Since this is so, the final sentence of the section of the encyclical cited above must be understood to mean that every act of marital intercourse must remain open to the transmission of life *when the possibility of communicating life to a new human being is present in the act itself.* It is obvious that it is not intended as a descriptive statement but as a *normative* judgment.

The Pope continues:

That teaching, often set forth by the magisterium, is founded on the inseparable connection, willed by God and unable to be broken by man on his own initiative, between the two meanings of the conjugal act: the unitive and the procreative. Indeed, by its intimate structure the conjugal act, while most closely uniting husband and wife, capacitates them for the generation of new human lives, according to laws inscribed in the very being of man and woman. By safeguarding both these essential aspects, the unitive and the procreative, the conjugal act preserves in its fullness the sense of the true mutual love and its ordination towards man's most high calling to parenthood. We believe that the men of our day are particularly capable of seizing the deeply reasonable and human character of this fundamental principle.

It is in fact justly observed that a conjugal act imposed upon one's partner without regard for his or her condition and lawful desires is not a true act of love, and therefore denies an exigency of right moral order in the relationships between husband and wife. Likewise, if they consider the matter, they must admit that an act of mutual love, which is detrimental to the faculty of propagating life, which God the creator of all has implanted in it according to special laws, is in contradiction to both the divine plan, according to whose norm matrimony has been instituted, and the will of the Author of human life. To use this divine gift destroying, even if only partially, its meaning and its purpose is to contradict the nature both of man and of woman and of their most intimate relationship, and therefore it is to contradict also the plan of God and His will. On the other hand, to make use of the gift of conjugal love while respecting the laws of the generative process means to acknowledge oneself not to be the arbiter of the sources of human life, but rather the minister of the design established by the Creator. In fact, just as man does not have unlimited dominion over his body in general, so also, with particular reason, he has no such dominion over his generative faculties as such, because of their intrinsic ordination towards raising up life, of which God is the principle.[23]

Pope Paul, in brief, sees the immorality of contraceptive intercourse in the fact that it necessarily negates, through human agency, the procreative dimension or meaning of human sexual intercourse and the relationship between this dimension and the unitive meaning or dimension of intercourse. His argument, basically, is that just as it is wrong to have intercourse that is destructive of love (intercourse that destroys the unitive meaning of this act), so it is wrong to have intercourse that is destructive of procreation. He also holds that the use of contraceptives constitutes an immoral exercise of our sewardship over our own body-persons.

The reasoning in Paul's encyclical has been seriously questioned. Even before the encyclical appeared, many Catholics, including prominent moral theologians, had argued that the opposition to contraceptive intercourse was predicated upon an outmoded notion of the natural law, which put excessive stress on the biological processes and the laws that regulate human conception. They agreed that the procreative and unitive dimensions of sexual intercourse are inherently related, but they argued that they are separable (as during specific periods of a woman's menstrual cycle) and that there are good reasons for separating them by human agency. The argument developed by those who opposed the traditional teaching of the Church foreshadowed the type of argument in the passage from Häring. The rationale for justifying contraception under specific circumstances was well summed up in the "Summary Document on the Morality of Birth Control," popularly known as the "majority report" of the special papal commission on the regulation of birth. The authors of this document declared that "when man intervenes in the procreative process, he does this with the intention of regulating and not excluding fertility. Then he unites the material finality toward fecundity which exists in intercourse with the formal finality of the person and renders the entire process 'human.' "[24]

According to the authors of this report, a contraceptive mentality must be avoided. This means that the marriage, as a whole, must be open to the transmission of life, but this does not require that every conjugal act within the marriage be open to procreation; acts that are infertile by intention or are rendered infertile by human agency are ordered to the expression of the couple's union in love, toward the unitive meaning of marital intercourse. Such contraceptive conjugal acts, therefore, cannot be judged moral or immoral in isolation from the total context of the marital union; rather, they derive their full moral quality from the fact that they are ordered to the fertility of the marriage relation as such. Such an understanding of human intervention in intercourse, it is argued, protects the good of procreation and recognizes that the procreative and unitive dimensions of sexual intercourse are inherently interrelated.[25]

The authors of this report also argued that the "true opposition" is not to be sought between material conformity to the physiological processes of nature and artificial intervention. It is only "natural" for man to use his intelligence and skill to control what is given by physical nature. The opposition is to be sought between one way of acting, which is contraceptive but respects the good of procreation and recognizes the inherent link between the unitive and procreative meanings of marital intercourse, and another way of acting, which is contraceptive and opposed to the good of procreation. The first type of contraception is morally justifiable whereas the latter is not.[26]

Put more briefly, the opposition to the teaching in *Humanae Vitae* is that the encyclical deems unnatural what many people consider to be a moral and natural function of human intelligence in man's endeavors to bring physical nature under intelligent control. As one writer put it, "Birth Control was for a very long time impeded by the physicalist ethic that left moral man at the mercy of his biology. He had no choice but to conform to the rhythms of his physical nature and to accept its determinations obediently. Only gradually did technological man discover that he was morally free to intervene creatively and to achieve birth control by choice."[27]

Before we offer critical observations about the line of argument that is advanced to justify contraceptive intercourse (and extended to justify eugenic sterilization), it is important to note areas of agreement between advocates of contraception and those who, like Paul VI, judge it to be inherently evil. First, both sides agree that there are many good, indeed compelling reasons why married couples ought not have more children, or even any children at all, as when there is an exceptionally high risk of passing on to a child a severely crippling genetic disease. Second, there is agreement that sexual intercourse between married persons can and ought to foster their love for one another and that it is not necessary that intercourse be fertile or there be procreative intent for it to be good and wonderful. There is no obligation that every act of intercourse between married couples result in the conception of a child; to the contrary, serious reasons can make the avoidance of conception morally obligatory.

With these observations as prologue, I propose to examine the argument that has been advanced to justify contraceptive intercourse and eugenic sterilization and I will conclude by offering further reflections on the question.

The argument for contraception and sterilization can be summed up by saying that these acts and practices are morally permissible because they (1) are well motivated and efficiently promote worthwhile goals, (2) need not repudiate the inherent interrelationship between the unitive and procreative meanings of marital intercourse but simply distinguish between specific acts of marital intercourse and the thrust or direction of marital life as a whole, and (3) represent rightful exercise of man's dominion over his body. (Häring justifies eugenic sterilization on *thera-peutic* grounds, as serving the health of the couple.)

With respect to the first point, it need only be said that good motives and good consequences do not, of themselves, justify the deeds we choose to do. If, however, one adopts this way of thinking about moral questions, he has already, in principle, justified *any* kind of human deed or act or practice. In other words, the first element of the argument, taken by itself, reflects a consequentialist mentality. As used by those who justify contraceptive intercourse and eugenic sterilization, it reflects "proportionate good" consequentialism, which most Roman Catholic writers who accept contraception and eugenic sterilization also accept because they believe a proportionate good is thereby served, namely, the unitive good of marital intercourse, and that this justifies the direct intention to destroy another good of marital intercourse, namely, the procreative good. This ethics has already been examined and rejected as incompatible with the ethics described in the Introduction.

The second element in the argument requires more extensive comment. It depends on a strangely reasoned distinction between a "contraceptive mentality" and specific acts of contraceptive intercourse for its validity. The authors of the majority report, Häring, and other Roman Catholic opponents of *Humanae Vitae* agree with the Pope that there is an inherent interrelationship between the procreative and unitive meanings of human sexual intercourse. They reject the separatist mentality (described in the previous chapter) and condemn as immoral a contraceptive, antiprocreative mentality, but contend that the choice to have contraceptive marital intercourse is not of necessity an indication of a contraceptive mentality.

I grant that a person's mentality, attitude, and identity may not be adequately reflected in an individual act, but there is a relationship between individual acts and a person's moral identity, which these authors seem to forget. There is a definite relationship inasmuch as we shape or "create" our moral identity by our willingness to choose to act in certain ways. For instance, I become an adulterer by being willing to choose to commit adultery. It is possible that I may not become fully identified as an adulterer by being willing to commit one act of adultery; this act may not be an expression of my personal being, so that in choosing to engage in it I may experience what St. Paul described so eloquently when he said he could not understand his actions and, instead of doing the good he wanted to do, did the evil that he hated (Rom 7:15–16). But if I continue to engage in acts of adultery I will become an adulterer, even if, paradoxically, I do not want to become one.

It is imperative in this connection to note that contraceptive intercourse, with pills, diaphragms, jellies, and so on, is by no means, if it is to effect the desired goal—preventing conception while permitting the genital expression of marital love—an isolated act. It demands a policy decision, the choice to adopt the *practice* of contraceptive intercourse for a prolonged period. It is therefore difficult to see how it is possible to choose this policy, to adopt this practice as a way of life, without taking on a "contraceptive mentality," whether one realizes that this is happening or not. The mentality imperceptibly becomes a dimension of one's existence, a part of one's "nature." A person might practice contraceptive intercourse and *say* that he does not have a contraceptive mentality, and he might believe this (perhaps because he really loves living children), but actions speak louder than words.

The distinction between a contraceptive mentality and contraceptive acts is, I believe, specious. Undoubtedly, those who propose it do so because they believe that contraceptive acts need not of necessity *proceed from* a contraceptive mentality, in which they are surely correct, but they fail to realize that the deliberate choice to act contraceptively imperceptibly *generates* a contraceptive mentality. I think this can be made clear in examples from other areas of life. Many persons sincerely believe they are not racist or anti-Semitic or alcoholic, and will vehemently deny it if they are accused of being so. But if these people habitually *act* as racists or anti-Semites or cannot go for a day without having a drink or two, they show through their actions that they are racist or anti-Semitic or alcoholic. Actions speak louder than words.

Thus the second key element in the argument to justify contraceptive intercourse and eugenic sterilization turns out to be very weak. It's like arguing that it is wrong to lead the life of a rapist but that an occasional act of rape (or indeed the practice of raping over a long period of time) is morally justifiable so long as some worthwhile good is achieved (perhaps psychotherapy in some situations) and the mindset or mentality of a rapist is avoided. The difficulty, of course, is that this mindset is inevitably acquired.

The third element in the argument needs careful assessment. It holds that these acts or practices are morally justifiable inasmuch as they represent rightful exercise of man's dominion over his body or legitimate human intervention into the course of nature. Thus the use of contraceptives and eugenic sterilization is justified on analogy to the use of drugs and surgery in other medical situations. Just as it is permissible for human beings to extract decayed teeth, to remove tonsils and appendices, to implant heart pacemakers and to transplant organs, so it is permissible to use a contraceptive pill or diaphragm or condom or whatever to render intercourse infertile—and ultimately to undergo a vasectomy or tubal ligation. Applied to preventing the birth of children who would be crippled by recessive genetic diseases, the argument would be that contraception and sterilization are a form of preventive medicine, but the analogy with therapeutic medical intervention must be questioned.

In warranted medical intervention a diseased organ or pathological disorder affects the human person—a condition that does not obtain in the use of contraceptives and sterilization. The "therapy" seems rather directed toward human desires, namely, to intercourse without risk of conception. But perhaps one could argue that in using contraceptives or undergoing sterilization for eugenic purposes there *is* a pathological condition, namely, recessive genes, and that although contraceptive devices and sterilization do not cure these genes, they prevent them from injuring future human beings. It is necessary to respond that there are realistic alternatives to preventing the harm that recessive genes may cause, namely, many natural methods of determining the infertile periods of woman and abstinence from sexual intercourse.

These alternatives need to be seriously considered, not only for moral reasons but for medical reasons as well, inasmuch as they do not pose the risks to the woman's health that contraceptives do (preeminently the pill) and they can be as effective as artificial means. Although it is common to dismiss rhythm sarcastically as "Vatican roulette," all natural methods of spacing children, as indicated for eugenic purposes, for forgoing the choice to have children of one's own, are quite effective.[28]

It is not proper to liken contraceptives and sterilization in rendering intercourse infertile to such medical interventions as the removal of a diseased tooth or organ to such technological interventions as damming rivers, digging tunnels, or irrigating deserts. The human body is not a part of the physical world over which man has been given stewardship; our bodies are not of a nature different from *human* nature. It is not as though a human being were a composite of an animal and a human nature, with human nature consisting in thought and free choice. A human being *is* an animal, though radically different from other animals. Our bodies, with their physiological and biological constitutive processes, are integrally human and their mutilation in contraception and sterilization[29] requires a genuinely therapeutic reason, as does the removal of a tooth. A latent dualism or angelism is discernible in the arguments advanced by many contemporary Roman Catholic moral theologians to justify contraception and sterilization.[30]

God has given us stewardship over creation and over our own persons. As his images, we participate in his providential rule over the universe and have the great gift of determining our lives through our own free choices. But God alone is the Lord of life and has total dominion over creation. As his stewards or vicars, we are to receive with love the gifts he has given us. Our bodies, our animality, are a good gift of God. Our procreative power, which ought never be degraded to a mere biological function, is a symbol of our likeness to him in our ability to bring life into existence and to communicate life and love to a new generation. Sterilization and contraception may be technologically efficient tools for coping with some agonizing human problems, but they represent a utilitarian manipulation of created reality, a pragmatic devaluing of our personal power to procreate. Genuine stewardship, which implies loving acceptance of the good gifts of creation, demands a more fitting response.

I appreciate the agonizing problems a married couple face who realize that they are carriers of a recessive genetic defect that could result in crippling their child, should they choose to have one of their own. But the agony they suffer is not different from that of other married couples who must, for various good reasons, avoid having more children. Such couples should be given detailed instruction in the best methods of natural family planning and should, as Christians, realize that there are millions of ways in which they can express their love for one another. If abstinence from sexual intercourse, even for prolonged periods, is the only moral alternative (though this can be seriously questioned), they should realize that this is required of them. They should also recognize that the conception and birth of a child who is handicapped by a recessive genetic disease is not the greatest tragedy in the world.

If voluntary contraception and sterilization were permissible and justifiable along the lines of the arguments advanced by Häring, it would also seem possible to justify *mandatory* sterilization in some situations. For instance, ought not feebleminded individuals, who are incapable of exercising responsibility over their actions, be sterilized for their own good and the good of society? In his provocative book, *Come, Let Us Play God,* Leroy Augenstein tells of a young girl with an IQ of 35 who married a "budding genius" with an IQ of 70. Augenstein had just delivered their ninth child, and the mean IQ of their older children was 50. In his view, this wife and her husband should have been sterilized, whether they consented or not, to prevent the birth of children with such low intelligence and the consequent cost to the community of caring for them for their lifetimes.[31]

Would it not be possible to argue that when persons are incapable of exercising responsibility over their actions and do not understand that sexual intercourse leads to the conception and birth of children, those who are in charge of these persons could give "proxy consent" for tubal ligations and vasectomies? One could make this argument, but its validity obviously depends on the prior justification of voluntary eugenic sterilization, and this, as we have seen, has not been validly made.

There are surely alternatives for preventing persons who are incapable of taking responsibility for their actions from engaging in activities that will result in human suffering and misery. Moreover, is it not arrogant to maintain that the life of an imbecile or moron is one of suffering and misery? If genuine human and Christian care is given to persons who are incapable of understanding their own activities, would not this care extend to helping them avoid situations in which pregnancy is likely to result?

Perhaps it would be economically and technologically efficient to sterilize certain classifications of persons, but economic and technological considerations are not sufficient. Mandatory or compulsive sterilization would certainly constitute invasion of a human being's physical, personal integrity; it would be a step toward looking at certain persons simply as parts in a whole and not as wholes within that whole; it would be an initial step on the slippery slopes of a consequentialistic ethics.

Therefore mandatory sterilization of the feebleminded and other handicapped persons is immoral, and it is better to accept the birth of children and their existence in the human community, even if feebleminded and afflicted, than do a deed that violates the integrity of persons and repudiates their moral worth.

Chapter 3

1. Herman Muller, "Genetic Progress by Voluntarily Conducted Germinal Choice," in *Man and His Future* (London: J. and A. Churchill, 1963).

2. H. Harris, "Predicting the long-term effects of treating inherited diseases: some comments," in *Patient, Doctor, Society: A Symposium of Introspections,* ed. Gordan McLachlan (New York and London: Oxford University Press, 1972), p. 21.

3. *Ibid.*

4. *Ibid.,* pp. 23–26.

5. Gerald Leach, *The Biocrats* (Baltimore: Pelican, 1972), p. 129.

6. W. French Anderson, "Genetic Therapy," in *The New Genetics and the Future of Man,* ed. Michael Hamilton (Grand Rapids: Eerdmans, 1972), p. 110.

7. J. Lederberg, testimony during House Appropriations Subcommittee hearings on 1971 budget appropriations for Departments of Labor and Health, Education, and Welfare, 91st Congress, 2nd session, part 7, *Congressional Record* (1971), p. 915.

8. Leach, *op. cit.*, p. 118.

9. *Ibid.*

10. Hudson Hoagland in a letter cited by Roger L. Shinn in *Soundings*, 52 (Fall 1969):305.

11. John Dedek, *Contemporary Medical Ethics* (New York: Sheed and Ward, 1975), p. 112.

12. *Ibid.*, p. 113.

13. That eugenic sterilization is inherently linked to contraception is demonstrated by Charles Curran in "Sterilization: Roman Catholic Theologies of," *Linacre Quarterly*, 40 (May 1973):97–108. This essay was reprinted in Curran's *New Perspectives in Moral Theology* (South Bend: Fides, 1975) under the title, "Sterilization: Exposition, Critique, and Refutation of Past Teaching." On this topic also see Charles McFadden, *The Dignity of Life* (Huntington, Ind.: Our Sunday Visitor Press, 1976), pp. 84–88, 222–230. Curran is in favor of contraception and eugenic sterilization for grave reasons, whereas McFadden argues against both as inherently evil.

14. On this see the encyclical of Pope Paul VI, *Humanae Vitae,* and *Ethical and Religious Directives for Catholic Hospitals,* released by diseases: some comments," in *Patient, Doctor, Society: A Symposium* United States Bishops' Conference in 1971. See also the "Letter on Direct Sterilization" (*Documentum circa sterilizationem in noso comus catholics*) of the Congregation for the Doctrine of the Faith, March 13, 1975, and printed in *Origins* (June 10, 1976):33, 35. See Richard A. McCormick's comments on the above report, "Sterilization and Theological Method," *Theological Studies* 37 (September, 1976):471–77. Also my critique, "Sterilization: Catholic Teaching and Catholic Practice," *Homiletic and Pastoral Review,* 77 (August-September, 1977).

15. Even Paul Ramsey, whom I consider to be one of the best Christian ethicists writing in English today, justifies contraception. See his *Fabricated Man* (New Haven: Yale University Press, 1971), pp. 33–34. Ramsey adopts the argument (described in my text) that makes a crucial distinction between a separatist *mentality* regarding the procreative and unitive meanings of marital intercourse and specific *acts* of contraceptive intercourse.

16. Bernard Häring, *Medical Ethics* (South Bend: Fides, 1972), pp. 90–91.

17. *Ibid.*

18. Curran, *loc. cit.* (n. 13 above).

19. Dedek, *op. cit.,* pp. 114–120.

20. *Ibid.*

21. On this consensus see, e.g., Robert Hoyt, ed., *The Birth Control Debate* (Kansas City, Mo.: National Catholic Reporter, 1969), pp. 19–20.

22. *Humanae Vitae,* par. 11.

23. *Ibid.,* pars. 12–13.

24. For the text of the "majority report" see Hoyt, *op. cit.,* pp. 70–71.

25. *Ibid.*

26. *Ibid.*

27. Daniel Maguire, "The Freedom to Die," in *New Theology No. 10,* ed. by Martin Marty and Dean Peerman (New York: Macmillan, 1973), p. 188.

28. It is very helpful to consult the thoroughly up-to-date and comprehensive work by John F. Kippley and Sheila Kippley, *The Art of Natural Family Planning* (Cincinnati: Couple to Couple League, 1975).

29. On the fact that contraception and sterilization involve mutilation see McFadden, *op. cit.,* pp. 222–230.

30. See my article "Sex, Love, and Procreation" in *Homiletic and Pastoral Review,* 76 (May 1976):10–29. Reprinted in the *Synthesis Series,* Franciscan Herald Press.

31. Leroy Augenstein, *Come, Let Us Play God* (New York: Harper & Row, 1969), p. 87.

4: Protecting the Human Genetic Pool (II): "Screening" Fetuses and Abortion

The "screening" of populations—married couples with family histories of genetic diseases, members of groups that are particularly susceptible to genetic diseases (e.g., Negroes to sickle-cell anemia, Jews from the Baltic Sea area to Tay-Sachs disease), children, and the unborn—to determine whether they are carriers of recessive genetic disorders has been proposed to help protect the human genetic pool by preventing the birth of children afflicted by crippling genetically-related diseases.

With respect to screening adult populations and even children with a view to educating and alerting them to the possibility of passing on crippling disorders, there are no overwhelming ethical dilemmas. (We shall return to this kind of screening in chapter 5, when we take up the question of genetic counseling.) It can be said, with Paul Ramsey, that "screening with a view to the prevention of conception seems clearly justified, if not indeed positively mandated. In this case, patients are given knowledge they need to know for 'responsible parenthood,' i.e., to embrace responsibility for not transmitting knowable defects to their children."[1] Such screening can serve an educative purpose, enabling persons to make their own responsible choices about having children of their own or, possibly, of entering marriage with certain kinds of persons.

Screening the unborn, however, raises very serious ethical problems. As currently practiced (e.g., when Tay-Sachs disease is suspected, when there is indication that a child may be afflicted with Down's syndrome, etc.), the procedure is to perform an amniocentesis on the pregnant mother. This involves removal of a small amount of amniotic fluid from the amnionic sac by a hollow needle; the fluid contains cells of the unborn child, and these can be subjected to chromosomal analysis. If a serious defect is discovered, the usually recommended procedure is to "terminate" the pregnancy by a "therapeutic abortion." Although, as one writer put it, "some people have strong moral objections to such a procedure, others feel that the suffering produced for the child, the mother, and the rest of the family by genetic defects is so great that any efforts toward prevention of defective babies is justified, including therapeutic abortion."[2]

Screening with a View to Abortion

Prescinding for the moment from the question of therapeutic abortion (to which we shall soon turn), we note that several observations about screening with a view to aborting fetuses with genetic defects are in order. It is obvious that most of those who advocate this procedure are not cold, ruthless, insensitive persons. They are motivated by compassion for people, for the suffering that human beings experience when genetically crippled children are born. They want to alleviate human misery. Through amniocentesis, followed by abortion, they seek to minimize suffering and maximize the good life—to bring about the greatest possible good for the greatest number of people.

However, in their desire to alleviate suffering, they have adopted a consequentialistic ethics that justifies human activities in terms of the good results these activities can bring about. Since this pragmatic way of approaching moral issues can justify anything on the grounds that the end justifies the means, it can justify amniocentesis and abortion as a morally right way of preventing human suffering. This ethics is obviously at variance with the ethics set forth in this work. The practice of screening the unborn with a view to aborting those who are found to be genetically crippled does an injustice to the "defective" unborn who will be aborted as a result, which will become clear later in this chapter. But even if we prescind from the morality of aborting "defective" fetuses, there are strong moral arguments against screening with a view to abortion.

First of all, as Ramsey develops in a striking way, screening the unborn is very poignant "because these patients do not suffer from a contagious disease, often their treatment is not in view, and a validly implied consent is therefore absent, and sometimes normals may be harmed by the screening or by its follow-up."[3] One of the problems is that of the "false positive," an unborn child who is falsely identified as genetically crippled. In their desire to make sure that the screening process identifies all who are genetically deficient, the physicians who engage in the practice believe, as one of them put it, that "the screening test must be oversensitive, so that it identifies all cases. There should be a number of false-positives, but no false-negatives."[4] In fact, "a test accurate 99.99 percent of the time for a disease occurring once in 20000 persons should find one 'false positive' for each one affected."[5] This means that those who advocate screening by amniocentesis, followed by abortion, are willing to abort, that is, cause the death of, an unborn child who does not suffer from any genetic defect. It is very much like operating on the wrong patient, only worse, for in operating on the wrong patient the intent is to cure that patient of a malady from which he or she is thought to be suffering, whereas in abortion the purpose is to eliminate the being in question from the human community. There is and must be, if amniocentesis with view toward abortion is resorted to, a *willingness* to do this; and this surely tells us something not at all pleasant about the practice.

Second, amniocentesis involves risks to the unborn child. Admittedly, the risks are statistically low—1 to 2 percent—but the damage that may be induced in the unborn child by amniocentesis is quite grave. In fact, we do not know, nor can we learn, the full range of harm that the procedure may entail. It must be argued, however, that a slight risk of grave damage is a grave risk.[6] And the risk is in no way connected with helping the being who supposedly is in need of therapy.

Third, the "therapy" for those who are identified by amniocentesis as afflicted with a genetic disease (whether they are in fact so afflicted or not) is abortion. But to call an abortion of this kind therapeutic is to misuse the word "therapeutic." As Norman Rosten noted, "We have only a handful of crucial words standing between light and darkness. To blur the meaning of even one is to hasten darkness. I suggest that we keep our eyes and minds on language as we would upon our sanity."[7] To consider abortion as a type of therapy for the unborn child who is crippled by a genetic disease is to misuse language. It may be therapeutic for human beings other than the fetus in question but it is hardly therapeutic for the fetus. It is like saying that execution is therapeutic for the criminal—only in this instance we are not dealing with anyone who has committed a crime, unless being afflicted with a genetic disease is to be considered a crime.

Moreover, in some families with living children who are afflicted with the genetic disorder there is a realization that the choice to use amniocentesis to determine whether a fetus is going to suffer similarly and the willingness to abort this fetus weakens the parental bond with the children already afflicted. The expectant mother senses "that an already affected child felt threatened by her visit to the [amniocentesis] center when she found him hiding in the closet upon returning."[8] This poignant fact has something of critical significance to tell us about the moral meaning of screening with a view to aborting an unborn child who is discovered to suffer from genetic disease.

Finally, something even more paradoxical seems to be involved. The purpose of aborting fetuses, discovered through amniocentesis to be suffering from genetically induced disorders, is to alleviate the human condition, to minimize suffering, and to maximize the "quality" of life. Yet, as Dr. Thomas Hilgers has noted, studies in Eastern European countries where abortion is widely practiced as a form of birth control have shown a dramatic rise in premature births among women who have previously undergone abortion. With the rise in premature deliveries comes a rise in the risk of grave impairments to newborn children by reason of their prematurity, with subsequent suffering and cost to the children, their parents, and society at large.[9] This startling fact should cause those who advocate screening and abortion as a way of coping with the problem of genetically crippled children to take pause and reflect on the matter.

Abortion

Although in this chapter we are principally interested in the abortion of fetuses thought to be suffering from crippling disorders caused by genetic defects as a way of protecting the human genetic pool, abortion itself is of such significance and so dramatically illumines our lives as moral beings that it will be worthwhile to examine the question in some depth. Therefore I propose (1) to set forth the teaching of the Roman Catholic Church on abortion and (2) to examine two critically important issues that are pertinent to the abortion controversy, namely, the status of fetal life and the conditions under which one human being may rightfully cause the death of another. The discussion will conclude with some reflections on the abortion of "defective" fetuses.

Teaching of the Roman Catholic Church

The official teaching of the Roman Catholic Church is that direct abortion is inherently and always wrong.[10] This teaching is reflected in many official documents of the recent past, and three may be cited as illustrative. In an address on October 29, 1951, Pius XII stated:

> The baby in the mother's womb has the right to life immediately from God. Hence there is no man, no human authority, no science, no medical, eugenic, social, economic or moral "indication" which can establish or grant a valid judicial ground for a direct deliberate disposition of an innocent human life, that is, a disposition which looks to its destruction either as an end or as a means to another end perhaps in itself not illicit. The baby, still not born, is a man in the same degree and for the same reason as the mother.[11]

The bishops assembled at the Second Vatican Council maintained that

> whatever is opposed to life itself, such as any type of murder, genocide, abortion, euthanasia, or willful self-

> destruction . . . are infamies indeed. They poison human
> society, but they do more harm to those who practice
> them than those who suffer from the injury.[12]

Finally, Paul VI declared in his encyclical of July 1968, on human life, that

> the direct interruption of generation already begun, and
> especially direct abortion, except if done for therapeutic
> reasons, must be entirely repudiated.[13]

Pius XII and Paul VI expressly stipulate that the morally proscribed act is *direct* abortion. The former explains in broad outline the difference between direct and indirect abortion (what Paul VI had in mind when he spoke of "therapeutic reasons") as follows:

> We have on purpose always used the expression *"direct*
> attack on the life of the innocent," *"direct* killing." For
> if, for instance, the safety of the life of the mother-to-be,
> independently of her pregnant condition, should urgently
> require a surgical operation or other therapeutic treat-
> ment, which would have as a side effect, in no way willed
> or intended yet inevitable, the death of the fetus, then
> such an act could not any longer be called a *direct* attack
> on innocent life. With these conditions, the operation,
> like other similar medical interventions, can be allowable,
> always assuming that a good of great worth, such as life,
> is at stake, and that it is not possible to delay until after
> the baby is born or to make use of some other effective
> remedy.[14]

From the foregoing the official teaching of the Roman Catholic Church should be clear. It is always morally wrong, deliberately and of set purpose, to destroy fetal life, that is, to commit an act of direct abortion, although under certain conditions therapeutic activities, directly aimed at saving the life of the mother-to-be, are permissible even if these activities result in, and are foreseen to result in, the death of the unborn child.

The basis of this teaching, as John T. Noonan, Jr.[15] (among others) has pointed out, is the dignity or sanctity of human life. The teaching is predicated upon the beliefs that fetal life is human life, that every human being is of equal worth, and that every human being is a being of moral worth, the bearer of rights that demand recognition and protection—of rights that are his because they are given by God and rooted in his humanity, not because they have been conferred upon him by society or because he has achieved something through his personal activity that gives him a claim to rights that others do not possess.

In his important essay, Noonan observed that "the teaching of a religious body may invoke revelation, claim authority, employ symbolism, which make the moral doctrine it teaches binding for believers in the religion but of academic concern to those outside its boundaries." Or it may, he continued, "embody insights, protect perceptions, exemplify values, which concern humanity."[16] The teaching of the Roman Catholic Church on abortion is of the latter variety, because abortion is *not* a *religious* question in any narrow sense. It deeply touches the meaning of human existence and the character of human existence as a moral existence. If abortion is a wrongful act, it is so not because it is judged to be so by a religious authority but because of what it means as a human deed.

Charles E. Curran has observed that the teaching of the Church on abortion "depends on two very important judgments: the judgment about when human life begins and the judgment about the solution of conflict situations involving the fetus and other values."[17] The first judgment of which Curran speaks is clear enough; by the second he has in mind the distinction between indirect and direct killing. Since both of these judgments are at the heart of the matter, we shall turn to them.

Status of Fetal Life

That the status of fetal life (I use this term in an inclusive manner to refer to the unborn organism from conception until birth)[18] is central to the abortion controversy was recognized by the Supreme Court of the United States in its decisions in *Roe* v. *Wade* and *Doe* v. *Bolton*. The court expressly declared that it had no intent to "resolve the difficult question of when life begins,"[19] yet the court in fact pronounced judgment on this difficult question inasmuch as it found that the fetus is not, prior to viability, a being to be protected and is, even after viability, only the "potentiality of human life" or "potential life."[20] Obviously, if the fetus is only "potential life" or the "potentiality of human life," it is not itself life. If a being is only potentially something, it is not what it can become. A young boy is a potential father, but he is not *now* a father, nor could he be only a *potential* father if in fact he were already a father. Thus one must conclude that the Supreme Court legalistically resolved the question of when life begins: it begins when one is born.[21] Indeed, the court stated that its decision in *Roe* v. *Wade* and *Doe* v. *Bolton* would have been different had it decided that the fetus is truly a human life.

There are many different attitudes toward the status of fetal life. They range from the view, expressed by Philip Wylie, that the fetus is "protoplasmic rubbish" or a "gobbet of meat"[22] to the views that it is simply "gametic materials" (Joseph Fletcher),[23] a "blueprint" (Garrett Hardin),[24] a "part of the mother" (Havelock Ellis),[25] to the views that, at some stage of its intrauterine development, it is alive and human though not the subject of protectable rights (Daniel Callahan and Michael Tooley)[26]—or that it is indeed an individual human being and a subject of protectable rights.[27]

The views of those who call the fetus "protoplasmic rubbish," "gametic materials," a "blueprint," or a "part of the mother" can be dismissed as mere rhetoric that has been falsified by uncontroverted scientific evidence. To designate the developing fetus as protoplasmic rubbish or gametic materials is obviously to express one's emotional reactions and to adopt a rhetorical ploy.

Fletcher, who in one context endorses abortion as a means of getting rid of "gametic materials," elsewhere admits that the fetus is alive and humanly alive. But he maintains that the fetus is humanly alive only from a *biological* perspective, which is insignificant, and that it is by no means "meaningfully" human.[28]

Hardin's contention that the fetus is a blueprint is simply that, a contention, and is easily refuted. Unlike a blueprint, which is not alive and is entitatively distinct from the finished building, the fetus *is* alive and there is continuity-in-being between the fetus, the newborn child, the adolescent, the adult, and the aging person.[29]

The claim that the fetus is part of the mother's body is falsified by the fact that the fetus is genetically distinct in every cell of its being from the mother. The developing fetus is not a mass of undifferentiated cells; it has its own structure and develops its own nervous, circulatory, respiratory, and digestive systems.[30]

The views of those who maintain that the fetus is not humanly alive from the beginning but *becomes* so at some later point or stage during its development require closer examination. Different authors, of course, assign different points in fetal development when the developing entity becomes a *human* being; so a degree of arbitrariness is involved—a significant matter that Ramsey brings out quite strikingly in one of his essays on abortion.[31] Many assign special significance to viability, but this is clearly no more than an expedient to deny human significance to fetal life. Germain Grisez, who has best summed up the reasons why viability is not a reasonable or intelligent point in development at which to assign humanity to the fetus, notes that many contemporaries suggest that abortion is morally justifiable as long as the unborn is not "viable." Their reason, evidently, is that prior to viability the fetus cannot live apart from the mother, whereas afterward it can, and the usual time suggested for determining whether a fetus is viable is the twenty-sixth or twenty-eighth week of gestation. Grisez then makes the following observations:

> The notion of "viability" defined in any such simple fashion is without biological and medical foundation. . . . The reason why is not difficult to discover. Dr. Carl L. Erhardt and his colleagues studied mortality among infants born in New York City, 1958–1961. In general, they discovered that neonatal mortality—that is, death within the first twenty-eight days after live birth—mounted steeply as the length of pregnancy shortened below thirty weeks and as the birth weight dropped below fifteen hundred grams (about three pounds, five ounces). But 45 percent of white and 58 percent of non-white babies born during the twenty-sixth or twenty-seventh weeks of pregnancy survived through the neonatal period. Even under twenty weeks of pregnancy, more than 20 percent of those born alive survived the neonatal period. From this study alone . . . it is clear that "viability" is relative and does not provide a clear mark of demarcation. Besides length of pregnancy, such factors as the weight and race of the fetus make a significant differ-

ence. Of course, beyond a certain point there are no survivors. However, this point, whatever it happens to be, also is relative to present methods of caring for the premature. With improved techniques and equipment, going beyond the incubator toward the artificial womb, probably the vast majority of fetuses could survive apart from their mothers after twelve or fourteen weeks of pregnancy.

Perhaps even more misleading than the factual oversimplification involved in the idea of "viability" is the assumption that ability to live independently is a suitable criterion of individual identity. Biologically this is certainly not true, for the fetus is genetically and functionally an individual from its beginning, but it is not capable of living independently until long after birth.[32]

The fetus, prior to viability, can be compared to a person who uses deep-sea diving equipment. He is viable so long as his lifeline is functioning properly, and his individual identity is obviously independent from those who monitor this equipment. If they choose to sever his lifeline, or inject saline solution into it, he will obviously die, as will a fetus in similar circumstances. But neither the fetus nor the diver is nonliving; each is living and viable, that is, capable of staying alive, so long as each is provided with the environment necessary for sustaining life.

Some authors, for example, Baruch Brody[33] (following a lead suggested by Callahan), propose that the fetus becomes human as its brain develops. This criterion for determining when a fetus (previously only potentially human) becomes human is suggested on an analogy to "irreversible brain death" in determining when a human being has ceased to exist. Although irreversible death of the brain, as evidenced by a series of criteria, including tests for receptivity and responsitivity, spontaneous movement, and reflex activity and confirmed by completely flat electroencephalographs, is *one* indication that a human being has ceased to exist,[34] using the brain as *the* criterion for determining when a human being has come into existence is a poor one, unless one is willing to identify the brain as *the* organ that makes a human being a human being. Acceptance of this criterion seems to be based on the supposition that the "mind" is the same as the "brain" and makes a human being a human being, that is, the capacity, even if undeveloped, to perform acts of understanding and choice.[35]

A living fetus, moreover, prior to the development of the brain, has the capacity *within itself* to develop a brain and perform the operations which require a brain as their physical substratum. Everyone knows that the living, developing fetus will *of itself, and in virtue of what it already is,* develop a brain if it is allowed to continue to exist. The capacity or potential for developing this organ is rooted in the fetus, in its actuality. Likewise, everyone knows that a human being who has died and whose "brain death" is one indication of his demise will never of himself develop a brain. Thus the supposed analogy is false and of no critical significance in determining when we have in our midst a living human being, a fellow word of God.

There are, I believe, only two "points" in the life of the fetus that ought to be given serious consideration for deciding when we have among us a member of our species, a living image of God: namely, conception-fertilization and segmentation-implantation. Before we look at these two points or stages of fetal life as criteria for determining the humanity of the fetus, however, it is pertinent to observe the presuppositions of those who (with Fletcher, Tooley, Callahan, and many others) are willing to grant that a fetus is a human being, a member of the human species (at least after some stage of fetal development), yet justify its abortion if its continuation in existence poses a serious threat to the happiness and well-being of others. (Brody, it must be noted, is not among this group; he strongly and ably argues against abortion once the humanity of the fetus has been achieved—in his view, with the emergence of the brain.) [36]

Michael Tooley has accurately stated the presupposition that is common to all these authors and to those who share their views about the justifiability of aborting fetuses, even when they are admittedly living human beings. The presupposition is that "membership in a species is of no moral significance."[37] This means that merely being a human being is not morally important; it is not sufficient to make a human being a bearer of rights, a being of moral worth. However, if being a human being is not of moral significance, what is? Apparently, only certain members of the human species have moral worth or moral significance for these authors—those who have become "meaningfully" human, by which is meant human beings who have, as Callahan puts it, "a developed capacity for reasoning, willing, desiring, and relating to others."[38] For these authors, in other words, humanity, in the sense that humanity is of moral significance, is an achievement, not an endowment. To be a human being for whom society should be concerned, one must do or be capable of doing something that will enhance or promote human welfare (e.g., being capable of entering into "meaningful" human relationships). There are, in other words, various tests, differently described by various authors in this group, that one must pass before he is entitled to be called a human being in a meaningful sense, in a morally significant sense.

This position is ethically warranted *only* if those who hold it are capable of showing conclusively that the moral significance of human beings (one of the crucial ways in which they differ from other animals) can ultimately be explained, fully and adequately, in terms of a difference in degree of development in human beings (or at least in *some* human beings, namely, those who have become beings of moral worth) when compared to other animals. It is *not* rooted in a human being's being a different *kind* of animal.

The Christian understanding of human beings (which I accept as the *true* understanding and capable of being defended by good philosophical arguments) is that a human being is a different *kind* of animal from all other animals and that, therefore, membership in the human species is itself a morally significant and decisive factor: human beings are beings of moral worth and are capable of becoming moral agents, not because of something they do or achieve but because of who they are.

The point I am trying to make can perhaps be seen more clearly in a passage from Mortimer Adler. According to Adler's philosophical analysis, if men differ from other animals only in degree, that is, by doing something that other animals do not do, but only because they have not attained the stage of development that men have attained, then

> those who now oppose injurious discrimination on the
> moral ground that all human beings, being equal in their
> humanity, should be treated equally in all those respects

> that concern their common humanity, would have no
> solid basis in fact to support their normative principle.
> A social and political ideal that has operated with revo-
> lutionary force in human history could be validly dis-
> missed as a hollow illusion that should become defunct.
> . . . We can now imagine a future state of affairs in
> which a new global division of mankind replaces all those
> old parochial divisions based upon race, nationality, or
> ethnic group . . . a division that separates the human
> elite at the top of the scale from the human scum at the
> bottom, a division based on accurate scientific measure-
> ment of human ability and achievement and one, there-
> fore, that is factually incontrovertible.[39]

Indeed, the moral reasoning described by Adler in this passage
is precisely the moral reasoning employed by the authors to whom
we have referred, who concede that the fetus, at least from some
point of fetal development, is a human being, a member of the
human species, but nonetheless claim that it is morally justifiable
to terminate its life when its continuation in existence poses
problems that conflict with the "interests" of human beings who
have achieved "meaningful" human existence.

But when does a human being, a member of the human species,
a fellow word of God, come into our midst? Earlier I said that
only two positions need seriously to be taken into account, conception-fertilization and segmentation-implantation. Before we
assess the validity of these positions, it is useful to look at some
of the consequences that would seem to follow if the fetus (or,
more specifically, the blastocyst) *becomes* human only at segmentation-implantation (a process that begins on the eighth day
after conception and is completed by the twelfth day) and is *not*
human prior to that time.

Although abortions are usually not sought until after a woman
is aware of her pregnancy (long after segmentation-implantation),
there would surely be a strenuous effort to develop new and
better techniques for detecting fertilized ova and preventing their
implantation. Again, many of the "contraceptives" in current
use, such as IUDs and the "morning-after pill," which are condemned by many as abortifacients, would be seen as "anti-im-
plantation" devices and the moral argument against their use
would be weakened (even though, as we have seen, strong moral

arguments would show that their use is wrong). In fact, one of the proponents of the segmentation-implantation criterion, James Diamond, M.D., suggests that the term "conception," in the sense of conception of a human being, be reserved to designate the segmentation-implantation process, and argues that efforts to prevent implantation should be regarded simply as "anti-conceptive" and not as abortifacient.[40] This shows that the question is quite serious.

The basic reason why some contemporary writers, among them Paul Ramsey (who is one of the strongest opponents of abortion)[41] and Charles Curran,[42] claim that segmentation-implantation can be used for determining when the developing entity becomes a human being is that this seems necessary to establish its *individuality* as a human being. This seems necessary inasmuch as, prior to this stage of development, the living entity that is brought into being at conception-fertilization can *divide* into identical twins, and it seems to be possible (verified in mice)[43] that *two* fertilized ova, prior to segmentation-implantation, can combine to form *one* individually implanted fetus.

These phenomena raise questions about the individuality of the pre-implanted fetus but are not a "decisive rebuttal that a human being comes into existence at fertilization-conception." We are dealing with a problem that has by no means been resolved but *can* be accounted for on the assumption (as we shall see, a well-founded assumption) that a new individual human being has come into existence at conception-fertilization.

To take identical twinning first. No one knows how twinning happens, but one of the most reasonable ways of explaining it is to liken it to asexual reproduction, or the mode whereby an amoeba can divide into two distinct amoebae.[44] In this view, one individuated entity, the so-called developing fertilized ovum (which is *no longer* an ovum but a living entity, genetically human in its identity and clearly individuated and differentiated from its parents), *continues in its own individuated life* and generates *another* being of the same nature as itself. Another explanation of identical twinning sees the individuated and developing pre-implanted fetus as ceasing to exist and giving birth, as it were, to two offspring similar to itself. In this view, the twins are the grandchildren of their parents and the children of the original entity that was brought into being at conception-fertilization.[45] The precise resolution of this problem awaits an answer, but these two possible explanations (in my opinion the first is more likely and seems more reasonable in the light of our biological knowledge of asexual reproduction) show that the phenomenon of twinning by no means forces one to the conclusion that an individual human being was *not* in our midst prior to segmentation-implantation. And we *know* that the individuality of the pre-implanted fetus, with respect to its parents, is established at conception-fertilization.

Both Curran and Ramsey accept the segmentation–implantation criterion for the beginning of individuated human life principally because they believe that the phenomenon of recombination or "mosaics" refutes the conception–fertilization position. Here it needs to be stressed that such recombination of two developing genetically human organisms has never been empirically observed. The fusion that occurs in the embryos of mice and that gives rise to the objection in the minds of such writers as Curran and Ramsey was brought about in laboratory conditions. Thomas J. Hilgers, M.D., recently stressed that the zona pellucida surrounds early human life, much like the shell of an egg. Just prior to implantation the blastocyst breaks out of the zona in order to accomplish implantation. B. Mintz, the scientist who achieved recombination in mouse embryos, herself recognized that the function of the zona pellucida is to *prevent* fusion of developing embryonic life. The fusion of mice embryos was not observed in nature but was achieved in laboratory experiments. Thus Hilgers concludes that fusion of such life, while perhaps theoretically possible, is extremely unlikely, and he cites the outstanding French geneticist, Jerome Lejune, "There is *no* evidence in man of recombination between two eggs to form one individual."[46]

Even were this phenomenon to occur, it would not of necessity refute the position that individual human beings come into existence at conception-fertilization. Grisez compares the phenomenon to grafting in plants. Granting the fact that we can graft two individuated plants into one new plant, this in no way demonstrates that the two plants were not alive and individuated prior to their fusion. Rather it is that prior to their fusion they did exist as separate individual plants. Similarly, the combining of two developing human embryos into one would simply mean that the two had ceased to be and that a new embryonic human being had come into existence.[47]

This leaves us with conception-fertilization as the moment or point when a new human being, a living image of God, a fellow word, a being of moral worth, comes into being. There are solid reasons for holding that this, in truth, is the time that we have in our midst a new human being. Reality-making or truth-making factors are pertinent here. As C. G. Goodhardt of the zoology department at Cambridge University remarked in an exchange with Malcolm Potts:

> Dr. Potts has argued that human development is a continuous process . . . and that it is in principle impossible to define when a new human individual comes into existence. May I with great respect suggest that this is a view which is contradicted by biological knowledge? For there is a real discontinuity at fertilization, or to be pedantic, at the "activation" of the ovum which is not necessarily always the same thing. This is the point after, but not before, it becomes capable of completing its development without any further stimulus from outside. Once activated, the organism will carry on its development until it dies. That is what most of us would have called the moment of conception, however else the British Council of Churches may now have decided to define the word. But whatever we call it, it occurs at a specific point in time, after, but not before which, development can proceed; and that is a real *discontinuity* marking the coming into existence of a new biological organism.[48]

The fetus—we are here concerned with the human fetus—is indisputably an entity that is living, that is individuated at least with respect to its parents, if not (prior to segmentation-implantation) with respect to any twins it might have, and that is identifiable as a human, as opposed to any other kind of living animal. There is an identity *in being* between the zygote, the fetus, the neonate, the child, the adolescent, the adult, the senior citizen. This new living entity is not potentially a human being but is *a human being with potential*, a potential it will develop if it is allowed to continue to be.[49] This entity does not, at some subsequent stage in its development, *acquire* human potential; it *already has* such potential, and it has this potential precisely because *it is the kind of being it is.* Its human potential is *real,* not an abstraction. From the time of conception-fertilization there is in our midst, though hidden from view, a new living entity that is identifiable as a member of tne human species and will develop all the properties or capacities that adult members of that species possess, not because the powers and capacities have been added to it from the outside but because they have been developed from within.[50]

The fetus—I am using this term in the broad sense, to designate the being that comes to be at conception-fertilization, implants in the uterus, and is viable in a uterine environment—is thus a member of the human species. Like all members of the human species, it is a being of moral worth, the bearer of rights that are to be recognized, respected, and protected by those members of the human species, fellow beings of moral worth, who have become (partially by virtue of the fact that they have been allowed to do so by others) moral beings or agents, capable of recognizing their fellow images of God, their fellow words, and of responding to them as they ought.

Since abortion destroys the life of a fetus, it can be justified only on the same moral grounds on which any other act that destroys human life is justifiable. But what are the reality-making or truth-making factors that are constitutive of a deadly deed that a human being may rightfully choose to do? The moral theory sketched briefly in the Introduction is fully compatible with a Christian understanding of human existence and the significance of human deeds. It is rooted in the thought of Thomas Aquinas[51] and is given contemporary expression by such writers as Germain Grisez and Paul Ramsey.[52] A human being may rightfully choose to do a deed that will cause the death of another human being only when his intent (biblically, his "heart," his moral person) is not to kill but to do a deed that is of itself an act of doing good. In such instances, the death that his act brings about is a foreseen, tragic, and terrible evil. The individual may willingly choose to do this deed only because it is in itself good. The evil caused, although foreseen, is not what the person may have intended nor is it the act's significance. Death in such instances may be permitted or allowed because there is some grave reason for doing the deed causative of it, but it is in no way the *means* to the good that the act accomplishes. To put it briefly, the "deadly" deed (i.e., the act causative of death) *is not an act of killing in the moral sense* of that term, but is rather an act of saving or protecting the good of life. Both the act and the intent of the actor are directed to the good inherent in and through the act, and no alternative acts could be chosen whereby this good could be protected and saved.[53]

Therefore, an act of abortion, insofar as it causes the death of a fetal human being, can be morally justified only on occasions (quite rare today) when the act itself is not ordered to the death of the fetal human being but is rather ordered of itself to protect the life of the mother. In such instances the death of the fetal human being is not intended. The death is not what the agent is intending to bring about, nor is this precisely what the act is bringing about. The death may be direct in an observable way, but the death is definitely not directly intended by the doer of the deed nor is the death of the fetus the moral meaning of the act. In such instances, abortion is not an act of feticide, because there are truth-making factors present and intelligibly discernible in the human act chosen that are not present in those acts of abortion in which the death of the fetus cannot not be intended.

Any abortion that is done precisely to bring about the death of the fetal human being, even if its death is reluctantly accepted, is not only tragic but immoral. Any abortion that is performed precisely so that the fetal human being will die is reprehensible. In such abortions the fetal human being, the child as yet unborn, is killed because it is not wanted for some reason or other, because its continued existence will conflict with the interests and needs of others and, perhaps, cause suffering. Therefore its death is directly willed and chosen.

To be willing to choose to do this kind of deed is to be willing to take on the moral identity of a killer, for the act is unquestionably an act of killing. But a Christian, indeed any human being, any word of God, ought not be willing to take on himself the identity of a killer, of one who sets his heart, however reluctantly, against the being of a fellow word of God. Since we make our moral identity by our willingness to choose to do things, we ought not be willing to choose to do acts that are acts of killing our fellow words of God.

Abortion of "Defective" Fetuses

When abortion is done to prevent the birth of fetal human beings who suffer from genetic defects, their death is obviously intended. The purpose of such abortions is to remove these human beings from the human community, to kill them, so that, perhaps, human suffering may be minimized. Although this kind of abortion is sometimes referred to as "therapeutic," to call it this is to misuse language. It does nothing to cure fetuses of the diseases they bear; death is a strange "therapy," a horrible "treatment." It may be "therapeutic" for the *desires* of human beings other than the fetal human beings in question, but it is by no means truly therapeutic.

It is instructive to cite the opinion of the Supreme Court of New Jersey in *Gleitman* v. *Cosgrove*. The parents of a boy, Jeffrey Gleitman, who was born congenitally defective in sight, hearing, and speech because his mother had contracted rubella during pregnancy, brought suit against the gynecologist-obstetrician, Cosgrove, in behalf of the boy on grounds that he had suffered a "wrongful birth." The court, in declaring against the Gleitmans, said:

> It is basic to the human condition to seek life and hold on to it however heavily burdened. If Jeffrey could have been asked as to whether his life should be snuffed out before his full term of gestation could run its course, our felt intuition of human nature tells us that he would almost surely have chosen life with defects against no life at all. "For the living there is hope, but for the dead there is none" (Thucydides). . . . *The right to life is inalienable in our society.* A court cannot say what defect should prevent an embryo from being allowed life. . . . Examples of famous persons who have had great achievements despite physical defects come readily to mind, and many of us can think of examples close to home. A child need not be perfect to have a worthwhile life. . . . The sanctity of the single human life is the decisive factor in

> this suit in tort. *Eugenic considerations are not control-*
> *ling. We are not here talking about the breeding of*
> *prize cattle.* It may have been easier for the mother and
> less expensive for the father to have terminated the life
> of their child while he was an embryo, but these alleged
> detriments cannot stand against the preciousness of the
> single human life to support a remedy in tort. . . . We
> firmly believe the right of their child to live is greater
> than and precludes their right not to endure emotional
> and financial injury.[54]

The great tragedy is that the ruling of the New Jersey Supreme Court, so eloquently expressed in 1967, was replaced by the folly of the Supreme Court of the United States in 1973.

A final comment bears repeating. The purpose of aborting physically or mentally defective fetuses is to help alleviate the human condition, to minimize suffering and to maximize the "quality" of life. But such abortions not only repudiate the sanctity of life, they also, paradoxically, contribute to the very problem they seek to remedy, as we have seen in studies that show a rise in premature delivery in women who have undergone abortions. With the rise in prematurity comes a rise in the incidence of grave impairments to the newborn, brought on by reason of premature delivery, with subsequent suffering and cost to the child, his parents, and society at large.

Of course it is possible, as Gerald Leach,[55] Michael Tooley[56] and an increasing number advocate, to give newborns a "trial period" of existence, so that they can be checked for defects and killed if the tests prove them to be "defective." This policy, which is consistent with the ethics of abortion and is seriously advocated today, tells us something about ourselves that is surely horrible and utterly opposed to a Christian understanding of what it means to be a human being.

These comments by James Schall in his excellent book, *Human Dignity and Human Numbers,* are worth pondering:

> Historically, it is of some importance to recall that the
> governmental origins of movements for the health and
> welfare of the poor and sick were found in religion, usual-
> ly Christianity, and gradually secularized. It was the be-
> lief that the deformed and the sick must be cared for that
> led to movements for their care and improvement. Even

more anciently, it was the Christian horror of infanticide
that led finally to the dropping of this commonly accepted practice. *What we are now beginning to witness is a
change in the fundamental belief that such a mission to
the weak and poor and deformed is worthwhile.* [Em-
phasis added.][57]

Chapter 4

1. Paul Ramsey, "Screening: An Ethicist's View," in *Ethical Issues
in Human Genetics,* ed. Bruce Hilton, Daniel Callahan, Maureen
Harris, Peter Condiffer, and Burton Berkley (New York: Plenum,
1973), p. 150.

2. W. French Anderson, "Genetic Therapy," in *The New Genetics
and the Future of Man,* ed. Michael Hamilton (Grand Rapids: Eerdmans, 1972), p. 116.

3. Ramsey, *art. cit.,* p. 151.

4. Charles A. Janeway, "Screening for Inherited Diseases: Editorial,"
New England Journal of Medicine, 284 (1972):787, cited in Ramsey,
art. cit., p. 152.

5. W. Eugene Know, "What's New in PKU," *New England Journal
of Medicine,* 283 (1970):1404, cited in Ramsey, *art. cit.,* p. 154.

6. See Ramsey, *art. cit.,* pp. 155–156.

7. Norman Rosten, *New York Times,* Mar. 19, 1970.

8. John Fletcher, "The Brink: The Parent-Child Bond in the
Genetic Revolution," *Theological Studies,* vol. 33 (September 1972):
470.

9. Thomas Hilgers, M.D., in Thomas Hilgers and John Horan, eds.,
Abortion and Social Justice (New York: Sheed and Ward, 1973), pp.
72, 313–315.

10. Competent presentations of the official teaching of the Roman
Catholic Church on abortion may be found in Germain Grisez, *Abor-
tion: The Myths, the Realities, and the Arguments* (New York: Cor-
pus, 1970), pp. 165–184, and in Richard A. McCormick, "Past Church
Teaching on Abortion," *Proceedings of the Twenty-third Annual
Convention of the Catholic Theological Society of America* (Yonkers,
N.Y.: CTSA, 1969), pp. 131–151.

11. *Acta Apostolicae Sedis,* 43 (1951):838–839.

12. "The Pastoral Constitution on the Church in the Modern
World" (*Gaudium et Spes*), par. 27, in *Documents of Vatican II,* ed.
Walter M. Abbott (New York: Guild Press, 1966), pp. 226–227.

13. *Humanae Vitae,* par. 14; *Acta Apostolicae Sedis,* 60 (1968):490.

14. *Discorsi e Radio-messagi di sua Santita Pio XII,* 6 (12 Nov. 1944):191–192, cited in Grisez, *op. cit.,* pp. 182–183.

15. John T. Noonan, Jr., "An Almost Absolute Value in History," in *The Morality of Abortion,* ed. John T. Noonan, Jr. (Cambridge, Mass.: Harvard University Press, 1970), pp. 1–59.

16. *Ibid.,* p. 3.

17. Charles E. Curran, "Abortion: Law and Morality in Recent Catholic Thought," *The Jurist,* 33 (1973):174–175.

18. A word about terminology is necessary. *Zygote* refers .to the unicellular organism brought into being when the woman's ovum is fertilized or "activated" by a man's sperm; *embryo* in the strict sense refers to the developing organism from implantation until the end of the sixth or eighth week of development; *fetus* in the strict sense refers to the developing entity from the sixth or eighth week of development until the end of the pregnancy. In ordinary language, *fetus* and *embryo* are used synonymously to refer to the developing being from the time of conception until birth.

19. Roe v. Wade, X, *United States Law Week,* 41 LW (1–23–73): 4227.

20. *Ibid.,* X, XI, *loc. cit.,* pp. 4228, 4229.

21. On this see the perceptive comments of John T. Noonan, Jr. in *National Catholic Reporter* of Feb. 3, 1973.

22. Philip Wylie, *The Magic Animal* (New York: Doubleday, 1968), p. 272. This is a particularly virulent passage, filled with invective against the notion of the sanctity of life.

23. Joseph Fletcher, "New Beginnings of Life," in *The New Genetics and the Future of Man,* pp. 76–91.

24. Garrett Hardin, "Abortion—or Compulsory Pregnancy?" *Journal of Marriage and the Family* (May 1968), p. 250.

25. Havelock Ellis, *Studies in the Psychology of Sex* (New York, 1924), 6:607.

26. Daniel Callahan, *Abortion: Law, Choice, and Morality* (New York: Doubleday, 1970), pp. 378–409; Michael Tooley, "Abortion and Infanticide," *Philosophy and Public Affairs,* 2 (Fall 1972):37–65.

27. Among authors who set forth and defend this view quite ably are Grisez, *op. cit.* (n. 10); Noonan, *op. cit.* (n. 15); and Robert and Mary Joyce, *Let Me Be Born* (Chicago: Franciscan Herald Press, 1971). This is also the position so well developed by Paul Ramsey in many articles, in particular "The Morality of Abortion," in *Moral Problems,*

ed. James Rachels (New York: Harper & Row, 1971), and "Abortion: A Review Article," *The Thomist,* 37 (January 1973):174–226.

28. In his *The Ethics of Genetic Control: Ending Reproductive Roulette* (New York: Doubleday Anchor, 1974), Fletcher quite frankly admits that the fetus is biologically a human entity, a living human being.

29. See Grisez's perceptive comments in *op. cit.,* pp. 275–276.

30. A good biological study that clearly falsifies the view that the fetus is a part of the mother's body is Roland Nardone's "The Nexus of Biology and the Abortion Issue," *The Jurist,* 33 (1973):153–161.

31. Paul Ramsey, "Reference Points in Deciding about Abortion," in Noonan, *op. cit.,* pp. 60–100; see also his "Feticide/Infanticide upon Request," *Child and Family,* 9 (Fall 1970):257–272.

32. Grisez, *op. cit.,* pp. 32–33.

33. Baruch Brody, *Abortion and the Sanctity of Human Life: A Philosophical View* (Cambridge, Mass.: MIT Press, 1975), pp. 100–115. It should be observed, to Brody's credit, that he holds that the fetus is, after the development of the brain, fully a human being in a morally significant sense, with a right to equal protection under law as another human being. Here he is unlike Callahan, who, although not fully accepting the possession of a "brain criterion" for humanity, clearly inclines to it. But it really does not make any difference for Callahan as far as moral significance goes, for the fetus is still not a "person" in any morally significant sense and nuanced judgments can still be made in "conflict" situations. A brilliant critique of Callahan is given by Ramsey in his *Thomist* article, cited above in n. 27.

34. On this Brody is very much worth consulting. See below, chapter 7, pp. 162–165.

35. This, in fact, seems to be Brody's presupposition. It is not at all uncommon today.

36. See Brody, *op. cit.,* pp. 116–132.

37. Tooley, *art. cit.* (n. 26), pp. 44, 48, 55.

38. Callahan, *op. cit.,* pp. 497f.

39. Mortimer Adler, *The Difference of Man and the Difference It Makes* (New York: Meridian, 1968), pp. 264–265.

40. James Diamond, "Abortion, Animation, and Biological Hominization," *Theological Studies,* 36 (June 1973):305–322. For an excellent refutation of Diamond's position see Patrick Coffey, "When Is Killing the Unborn a Homicidal Action?" *Linacre Quarterly,* 43 (May 1976):85–93.

41. Ramsey accepts the implantation-segmentation criterion in his *Thomist* article, cited above (n. 27).

42. Curran accepts the segmentation-implantation criterion in the *Jurist* article cited above (n. 17). Unlike Ramsey, who holds that it is never morally permissible to kill the fetus after implantation unless this is "indirect," however, Curran will justify direct abortion if there is some commensurate good to be achieved.

43. Beatrice Mintz, "Experimental Genetic Mosaicism in the Mouse," *Ciba Foundation Symposium: Preimplantation Stages of Pregnancy,* pp. 194–207.

44. Brody, *op. cit.*, pp. 82ff., offers a good critique. See also Grisez, *op. cit.*, pp. 24–27. On this entire subject see Benedict Ashley O.P., in Albert Moraczewski O.P. and Donald McCarthy, eds., *An Ethical Evaluation of Fetal Experimentation* (St. Louis: Pope John XII Center, 1976), appendix.

45. See Grisez, pp. 24–27.

46. Thomas J. Hilgers, M. D., "Human Reproduction: Three Issues for the Moral Theologians," *Theological Studies* 38 (1977):136-52.

47. Grisez, *op. cit.*, pp. 27–28.

48. C. B. Goodhardt, "Reply to Dr. Potts," in *Biology and Ethics,* ed. F. C. Ebling (New York: Academic Press, 1969), pp. 101–103.

49. The Joyces, in the book cited above (n. 27), develop this thought very effectively.

50. On this see Francis Wade, "Potentiality in the Abortion Discussion," *Review of Metaphysics* (December 1975).

51. Thomas Aquinas did hold that one could rightfully intend the death of another human being if that human being were a criminal or a sinner. In other words, he justified capital punishment and the directly intended killing of those who were attacking innocent parties by public authority (cf. *Summa Theologiae*, 2–2,64, articles 1 through 6. But Germain Grisez has analyzed these texts of Aquinas (cf. *Abortion. . . . ,* pp. 323–325) and Aquinas is really being inconsistent with his own principles regarding the dignity of the human person and the value of life in justifying the direct intent to kill criminals and sinners. The principal point, so far as our present discussion is concerned, is that Aquinas held that it was morally wrong to intend to kill, i.e., to intend directly the death of, an innocent human being. Nonetheless he argued, in *Summa Theologiae*, 2–2, 64, 7, that not all the effects of actions that we freely choose to do come equally into the scope of our intentionality. Thus we may freely choose to defend ourselves (or others) from attack even if we foresee that the assailant will be killed as a result of our act of self-defense. In such in-

stances, the death of the other person is itself not directly intended, nor is it precisely the direct object of the deed.

This is not the place to discuss further this issue in Aquinas. Readers may note that the question is at the heart of the moral reasoning in the principle of double effect, and it is precisely in endeavoring to understand what this principle means that both Grisez and Ramsey appeal to the thought of Aquinas in *Summa Theologiae*, 2–2, 64, 7. A short study of this principle, along with the question of its origin in the thought of Aquinas and its interpretation by modern writers, is given in my "Double Effect, Principle of," *Encyclopedia of Bioethics,* ed. Warren T. Reich (New York: Macmillan-Free Press, 1977).

52. For Grisez see *op. cit.,* pp. 321–346 and his more extended discussion in "Toward a Consistent Natural-Law Ethics of Killing," *American Journal of Jurisprudence* 15 (1970): 64–96. For Ramsey see in particular his essay, "Abortion: A Review Article," *The Thomist* 37 (January 1973): 174–226. There are indeed differences between Grisez and Ramsey. Still in my judgment the agreement between the two is most significant, along with the explicit reference that both make to the teaching set forth by Aquinas. With Grisez and Aquinas Ramsey agrees that "any killing of man by man must be 'indirect'" (p. 220), if it is to be morally justifiable. This is precisely the position taken here.

53. It is evident that the line of thought developed here is dependent on the rule or principle of double effect. Readers will find this principle defended and interpreted by Grisez and Ramsey in the articles and works cited. I have commented at more length on the relevance of this principle to abortion in "Abortion and Man's Moral Being," in *Abortion: Pro and Con,* ed. Robert Perkins (Cambridge, Mass.: Schenkman, 1974), pp. 13–35.

I realize that the position taken here is in some way a departure from positions officially taken by the magisterium of the Church, as illustrated in the Vatican document on procured abortions. But the major point is that an abortion, to be morally justifiable, must be "indirect," in the sense that the act is not as such an act of feticide but one of saving life, in which the death of the fetus is not properly intended. The Vatican documents reflect an understanding of the rule or principle of double effect that was common for many centuries, and this understanding quite properly was concerned to limit the evil that one could rightfully do in the pursuit of good.

54. 49 NJ 22, 227 A.2d 689 (1967) 693.

55. Gerald Leach, *The Biocrats* (Baltimore: Penguin, 1972), pp. 201–205.

56. Tooley, *art. cit.* (n. 26 above).

57. James Schall, *Human Numbers and Human Dignity* (New York: Alba House, 1971), p. 65, n. 16.

5: Protecting the Human Genetic Pool (III): Genetic Therapy, Genetic Counseling, and Responsible Family Planning

The more one knows, the greater moral responsibility he has, simply because of his cognitive awareness of human needs and the requirements of justice.[1] Since we know that there is a serious problem concerning the genetic future of the human race and why some children are born with terribly crippling disorders, caused by recessive genetic or chromosomal deficiencies,[2] there is an obligation for the present generation of human beings to minimize these dangers and to prevent, so far as possible and by means or deeds that are morally upright, the birth of children who may be seriously harmed by reason of their inheritance.

In the previous chapters we looked at some of the means proposed to achieve this goal and rejected them insofar as they cannot be reconciled with a love for the whole range of the human good, a created participation in the *summum bonum*, God himself. It must be recognized that the means already examined (e.g., sterilization of persons who are known to be carriers of recessive genes or chromosomally induced diseases and abortion of unborn children who are likely to be the victims of such diseases) may be efficient techniques for achieving this goal—although this can be seriously questioned.[3] But our concern is to discover the inherent meaning of the means, i.e., the acts, proposed; we want to know what willingness to choose them says about ourselves as responsible moral persons and as a society. And it is for this reason that these proposed means have been rejected. Still, their rejection does not leave us powerless, unable to cope intelligently with the very serious problem at hand. Our purpose now is to examine alternatives and reflect upon them. Three in particular merit close examination: (1) genetic therapy, (2) genetic counseling, and (3) responsible family planning.

Genetic Therapy

Genetic therapy (also called genetic surgery, nanosurgery, or microsurgery) has been defined by W. French Anderson, head of the section on human biochemistry, molecular disease branch of the National Heart and Lung Institute of the National Institutes of Health, as "the attempt to treat hereditary diseases by influencing the genes directly."[4] It is possible, at least in theory, for us to make this attempt because of breakthroughs in molecular biology, particularly the discovery that the DNA strands in our cells contain the "genetic language" of our body-persons.

The genetic language is made up of the linear sequence of only four types of nucleotides that are found in DNA. These four "letters" of the DNA "alphabet" are: adenine (A), cytosine (C), guanine (G), and thymine (T). Each of these is a specific chemical nucleotide, composed of carbon, nitrogen, oxygen, and hydrogen. "Words" are constructed, geneticists tell us, of three (and only three) "letters." For example, GCA is a code word in the DNA. Since four code letters, taken any three at a time, result in sixty-four possible combinations, there are sixty-four genetic code words, each with a specific meaning.

Geneticists now know a good deal about this "language" of our bodies. They realize that the substitution of one "letter" for another can cause a cell not to produce a given enzyme or protein that is essential for the normal functioning of the organism. *If it were possible to insert the right letter into the code word, to replace one that is "incorrect," it should be possible to correct a particular defect* (e.g., the failure, in those suffering from phenylketonuria, to convert the phenylanaline in their food to tyrosine) . Theoretically, this could be done in two different ways, by *transduction* and *transformation*. As Anderson describes them, the procedures would operate as follows:

> The most satisfactory treatment for a patient suffering a genetic defect would be actual correction of the genetic material itself. In bacteria it is now a routine laboratory procedure to correct genetic defects by altering the DNA of the bacterial cell. This is accomplished in one of two ways. In one method, pure DNA which carries the desired gene is given to the cell. A small percentage of cells incorporate the new genes into their gene pool. This process is called transformation. A second method is the use of carrier virus particles. The desired gene is attached to a nonpathogenic virus particle which then carries the gene into the cell where it is incorporated into the cell's genetic pool. This process is called transduction. Extension of these commonplace bacterial procedures to human cells is theoretically feasible.[5]

What can be said about this? If the procedures are genuinely *therapeutic,* that is, designed to correct a malady from which an individual human being is suffering, and if they offer some reasonable hope of success, there would seem to be no moral problem with their use that is different in kind from other problems associated with therapeutic practices in medicine.

But there is great need to specify what Anderson means by "genetic material" and by "altering the gene directly." Are we speaking about the gametic cells of prospective parents who carry an inheritable disease but are not themselves afflicted by it, the developing zygote, blastocyst, embryo, fetus, or what? If "surgery" is directed toward correcting "errors" in the gametic cells of prospective parents, are we really treating a patient? Or are we not as Paul Ramsey has observed,[6] treating a *desire* of prospective parents for a healthy child, and in doing this are we not perhaps taking unwarranted risks in behalf of the child who may be conceived? Anderson admits: "It is not known, *nor can it clearly be tested* [author's emphasis], what effect any virus, believed to be nonpathogenic or not, will have on the gene pool. . . . We may have the ability to manipulate genes long before we know whether it is safe to do so."[7]

Genetic surgery performed on the germinal cells of prospective parents may actually cause greater harm to the child-to-be than might be induced by the genetically caused disease which the surgery is intended to prevent. This, at any rate, seems to be probable in the present state of scientific development. There would thus be no proportionality for undertaking such surgery at the present time. Thus this type of genetic surgery would seem to be subject here and now to the same kind of rejection merited by *in vitro* fertilization. In the future, after sufficient experimentation has been done on higher mammals, such genetic surgery may be justifiable when *positively induced* damage by the surgery on the child-to-be can be *reasonably* excluded. The purpose of the surgery will *then* be preventively therapeutic for the child in question, and not simply for the desires of prospective parents. And the situation will differ morally from that of *in vitro* fertilization insofar as there is reason to fear that a child will be genetically crippled *unless* preventive surgery is done, whereas with respect to *in vitro* fertilization this danger is absent and the whole purpose is simply to treat the desires of prospective parents for a child of their own. If positively induced damage can be reasonably excluded, any damage caused would be proportionate and in itself not intended. Moreover, the probability that the surgery would do more good than harm would satisfy the requirement of proportionality.

If genetic surgery is performed on specific cells of a person afflicted with a genetically caused malady, it might be considered experimental therapy and would therefore be in principle justifiable. But up to the present, so far as I know, this is not possible. The only recorded instance of surgery of this kind involved two German sisters who suffer from argenisia. There is a real possibility that the virus that carried the "corrective" genetic code in this instance (the Shoppe virus) may be capable of correcting the mistake in the code that is responsible for the disease. The virus, as reported by Anderson,[8] was given to the two girls afflicted with the disease, one aged 14, the other 7. But, as Ramsey noted,[9] this virus is also known to be pathogenic, for it can cause cancer in humans. In addition, the 14-year-old sister had been so crippled by the disease that the researchers knew beforehand that there was no real possibility that the injection of the virus could be of benefit *for her*. Thus she was used as an experimental subject, and the pertinent facts indicate that her parents were not adequately informed about the nature of the experiment to give reasonably informed consent for a therapeutic experiment. Hence this example of genetic surgery was *not* morally justifiable, although in principle it may be possible for surgery of this kind, if performed on specific cells of persons afflicted with hereditary diseases, to be morally justifiable.

At the present state of scientific knowledge, it seems the best way for genetic surgery to go in the future is toward correcting genetic disorders in the cells of afflicted persons by "growing" entirely new organs and substituting them for organs that malfunction by reason of the cellular genetic code. Thus it might be possible to "grow" a new liver or pancreas or other organ for persons suffering from phenylketonuria or diabetes or other genetically induced diseases. Gerald Leach, citing Dr. Edward Tatum, describes this kind of gene therapy:

> The first successful genetic engineering will be done with the patient's own cells, for example, liver cells, grown in culture. The desired new gene will be introduced . . . and the rare cell with the desired change will then be selected, grown in a mass culture, and reimplanted in the patient's liver. Re-programming cells in this way could become an important tool for treating genetic defects. For example, by reprogramming the liver cells of a phenylketonuric child, one might give him a normal set of liver enzymes that would effect a total, permanent cure for his disease.[10]

This type of gene surgery does not pose any serious moral problems and it is the area in which research ought to be directed, for it offers reasonable grounds for success and does not take unnecessary risks on behalf of populations yet to be. It is a form of surgery ordered to the therapeutic good of real patients. It is also a type of experimentation that is genuinely therapeutic and for which reasonably informed and free consent can be requested, and for which, too, proxy consent is justified. The difficulty, however, is that it does not treat the genetic causes of the disease in question, for the germ cells of the afflicted persons would still seem to carry the recessive genes responsible for the deficiency and would be passed on to future generations.

Genetic Counseling

Genetic counseling is a growing area of contemporary medicine.[11] As currently practiced, such counseling includes recommendations for the sterilization of persons who discover that they are carriers of recessive genetic or chromosomal disorders, for amniocentesis followed by abortion, and for recourse to donor insemination. These practices are morally repugnant for reasons discussed in previous chapters. But genetic counseling is not limited to such suggestions. As such, genetic counseling ought to be a part of human education, and in particular it ought to be included in marriage preparation programs. In fact, it is becoming possible to screen individuals, long before they contemplate marriage, for various kinds of genetic defects, and it would seem that screening populations who are subject to certain types of serious genetically induced diseases would be an act of moral responsibility for it would give them important knowledge to take into account in planning their future. Proper counseling could forewarn particular persons that they ought to have a proper concern for the genetic well-being of a future generation of human beings and that, possibly, they ought not contemplate marrying persons who are, like them, carriers of particular genetic defects but rather seek, as the one with whom they will choose to share their life and communicate life and love to a new generation, a person who is genetically compatible.

The rules of many societies (including the community of the Church) concerning marriage between close relatives seem to have been prompted by a proper concern for the procreative good, inasmuch as experience had shown there is greater likelihood of children who might be crippled if their parents are closely related than if this were not the case. I believe that this experience has been deepened and broadened by our current knowledge of the *causes* of some very crippling hereditary disorders. Thus it may well be an act of moral responsibility to proscribe marriage within certain degrees of "congeniality," if this term may be used, as well as within certain degrees of consanguinity. Education with these thoughts in mind is surely a part of responsible genetic counseling. It does not issue in a demand for sterilization or "therapeutic" abortion of defective children, and it can be of service in halting the deterioration of the human genetic pool.

Responsible Family Planning

When married persons discover that they are carriers of serious genetic disorders, they have a moral responsibility to think seriously about exercising their procreative powers and having children of their own. The decision *not* to have children of their own can be a good moral decision, and perhaps obligatory. A husband and wife who come to this decision discover a real cross in their lives; they are confronted with tragedy and experience real suffering.

In our society there is a serious temptation even for right-thinking persons, confronted with this decision, to conclude that they can resort to sterilization or other contraceptive techniques, and it can be understood why such persons may reach this conclusion. Still, I believe that sterilization and other types of contraception, and of course "therapeutic" abortion, are not truly responsible human ways of coping with this human problem, and I hope that the arguments advanced in previous chapters have adequately given the reasons for this belief.

Wives and husbands who find themselves in this situation are in many ways placed in the same agonizing situation as wives and husbands who cannot, for other serious reasons, responsibly allow a pregnancy to occur. These people still have the obligation to foster their love for one another, to love even as they have been and are loved, and they will long at times to express their love for one another in genital intercourse. These persons ought carefully to investigate the many forms of natural family planning that are currently available,[12] particularly when, too often, such methods of responsible family planning are rejected out of hand as unreliable or ineffective. They must also learn how to express their affection for one another in other ways, sexually but non-genitally.[13]

It is not my purpose to describe the various types of natural family planning, such as the Billings or the mucus method, etc., inasmuch as other works describe them in detail,[14] but it is important to offer some reflections on the moral question at stake. Thus I should like to show that there is a real difference between contraceptive intercourse as a way or means of preventing conception and the practice of periodic, even prolonged abstinence from sexual intercourse and, second, to comment on the opinion, advanced by Bernard Häring, that rhythm and other forms of natural family planning lead to an increase in spontaneous abortions in early pregnancy and to an increase in crippled children as a result of "aging" gametic cells. I believe that previous discussions have shown why contraceptive intercourse and sterilization are pragmatic devaluings of the procreative meaning of marital intercourse; hence in the discussion to follow I will not repeat material already considered.

Contraceptive Intercourse vs. Periodic Abstinence

It is very important to see the difference between contraceptive intercourse and periodic abstinence as means of exercising responsible parenthood, precisely because so many people can see no difference between them, including prominent theologians. In fact, many regard rhythm, which they erroneously believe is the only type of natural family planning, as an "unnatural" and "insensitive" way of coping with the serious problems that married persons encounter in their endeavor to exercise parenthood responsibly, especially when a husband and wife discover they are bearers of a serious genetic disorder and there is a serious risk that any child they conceive may be crippled by it and suffer terribly as a result. Indeed, many Roman Catholic theologians, including such important figures as Bernard Häring[15] and James Burtchaell,[16] argue that contraception is morally justifiable precisely because rhythm or periodic continence has been judged by the magisterium of the Church to be morally acceptable, and for them this is simply one type of "contraception."

Those who believe that regulating conception through periodic abstinence and through contraceptive intercourse are morally the same frequently reach this conclusion because (a) the motives behind both modes of human activity are the same and (b) both practices lead to the same result, avoidance of conception.[17]

It can readily be granted that the *motives* of a couple who seek to avoid pregnancy through contraceptive intercourse and of a couple who seek to do so through periodic abstinence from marital relations may well be the same and may well be good. When the motivations for avoiding conception are good, as they are for married couples who do not wish to take an irresponsible chance of inflicting harm on a child-to-be because they are carriers of a crippling hereditary disease, we can say that persons who choose contraceptive intercourse and persons who choose periodic abstinence equally *mean* well.[18] But this is not the only or, indeed, the morally decisive consideration.

Motives and their meanings are one thing, whereas the acts one chooses to realize his motives are another. There is, of course, an interrelationship between motive and act, but it is necessary to distinguish between them,[19] and the major reason why we are interested in discovering the meaning of the acts we choose to do is that they tell us about ourselves and the kind of persons we are. They disclose or reveal our moral identity, and through our willingness to do them we make or shape our identity as moral beings.[20] This means that a well-motivated person may choose to do a deed he really ought not choose to do. He means well, but the "word" he speaks or utters through his act is ill chosen and speaks a language different from that spoken by his motives.

Let me illustrate this by considering the acts we may choose to do to express our love and compassion (our motives) for a pregnant woman who knows that her child may be crippled because she was afflicted by rubella during her pregnancy. We may, to manifest our loving compassion, urge her to have an abortion as a way of easing her pain and suffering. Our act is morally well motivated, for we choose the abortion not because we hate the unborn child but because we care for the mother and want to prevent human suffering, including the suffering the child will endure. But the act is an act of abortion, of fetal euthanasia. It has an intentionality and thrust that we cannot

not intend, and this intentionality and thrust (what St. Thomas referred to as the "matter" of the act)[21] give it a meaning or intelligibility that cannot be taken away or changed by our motives. And this meaning or intelligibility has something to say about our moral identity. Alternatively, to express our loving concern for the woman and her unborn child, we may choose to give her the strength to bear her child and to help her in caring for him. The motives that prompt both deeds may be the same but the acts that we freely choose to do to realize these motives are quite different in kind.

The same is true with respect to contraceptive intercourse and periodic abstinence from conjugal relations as acts that are freely chosen in order to be responsive to parental obligations. They are different kinds of acts, subject to different moral evaluations—and we have already evaluated the *meaning* of contraceptive intercourse.

The fact that both acts have the same result, namely, avoidance of pregnancy, is not the morally decisive factor. Our acts indeed *get things done*, that is, have results, but their moral meaning is not to be identified with their consequences. For in addition to getting things done, our acts *get things said,* and what they say is of crucial moral significance.[22] We can get the same thing done through quite different actions, and while the thing we get done may be very good, the act through which it is done may be very bad. For example, I may wish to enhance human knowledge and bring benefits to great numbers of people by performing an experiment with the help of volunteers. But this tells me nothing about the *nature* of the experiment (the act), and it may well be that one kind of experiment to secure this good is a good experiment whereas another kind is evil.

That there is a real difference between contraceptive intercourse and periodic abstinence as human acts, freely chosen as ways of exercising parental obligations, is demonstrable. In contraceptive intercourse there is, as it were, a double-barrelled choice: one chooses (a) to have sexual relations and (b) to destroy whatever procreative power there may be in those relations. Contraceptive intercourse is not only *non*procreative intercourse but *anti*procreative intercourse. One element of human choice in contraceptive intercourse is the direct intention to render impotent the procreative power of the human person, to inhibit this human power at least for the time at which intercourse is chosen. It is a choice to reject this aspect of our human personhood.

Persons who choose to exercise parental responsibilities through periodic abstinence choose to do something quite different from those who choose to have contraceptive sexual relations. The former choose, first of all, *not* to have conjugal relations if there is some probability that conception may result. They choose this not because they regard such relations as wrong; quite to the contrary, they recognize that conjugal relations are goods of the highest order, worthy of human love and respect, for they are meant to be expressions of the love they have for one another. Rather, they choose to forego this very great good, here and now, because they realize that (a) it would be irresponsible for them to have relations if conception is probable, because of a serious moral obligation to avoid pregnancy, and (b) were they to choose to have conjugal relations here and now and avoid the possibility of conception-pregnancy by contraceptive, antiprocreative means, they would be repudiating their gift of procreativity and hence responding negatively to a great human good.

There is, then, a real difference between contraceptive intercourse and periodic abstinence from intercourse as acts or means of exercising parental responsibilities. Obviously, were couples to choose not to have conjugal relations because they consider such relations dirty, vile, or to be "used" only for the generation of children or the avoidance of fornication, then the choice to abstain from marital relations would be immorally motivated and would amount to repudiation of the great good of marital intercourse. Similarly, persons could seek to avoid the conception of children by periodically abstaining from marital intercourse because of selfishness and unwillingness to share their lives and love with a future generation of human beings. If this were the case, it would be a wrongly motivated way of exercising parental responsibilities. It would express the mentality of "technical virgins," who want to know how far they can go without committing sin but whose minds are quite opposed to those of persons whose hearts are set on the good and who are open to its realization. It is a form of Pharisaism.

Thus periodic abstinence *can* be wrongly motivated, but persons who choose to abstain periodically from marital intercourse are not necessarily wrongly motivated. Since abstinence from marital relations is not in itself or inherently wrong, the choice to do so for morally good reasons cannot be wrong.

Nor is there anything wrong if married persons choose to have relations during infertile periods. They have the right to express their love for one another through the marital act so long as there are no morally compelling reasons for not doing so. In choosing to have marital relations during the infertile periods, a married couple in no way of necessity rejects or repudiates the procreative good of human sexuality and marriage or their own procreative powers. They choose to be *non*procreative but they do not choose to be *anti*procreative.

An analogy may be useful here. For a long time theologians, under the influence of St. Augustine, who articulated what could be called an exclusively procreative understanding of human sexuality,[23] justified marital intercourse only for the purpose of procreation, or, as a concession to human weakness caused by sin, for avoiding fornication. They failed to recognize the unitive good of human sexuality and marital intercourse, and they rejected marital intercourse for the pleasure of it. It took a long time for theologians (and others) to recognize that marital relations can serve other valid human goods besides procreation.[24]

It is surely wrong for married couples to be *anti*unitive in the marital act—which Pope Paul VI clearly recognized in *Humanae Vitae*[25]—but it is not necessary, though it is highly desirable, for a married couple *explicitly* to intend their act of marital intercourse to be an expression of their deepest love for one another in order for it to be a good moral act. They may choose to have relations simply for the fun of it, without explicitly intending either children or expression of their deepest love for one another. It is wrong for them explicitly to intend it to be *anti*unitive, a repudiation of the unitive good of sexuality and marital intercourse, or to intend it to be *anti*procreative, a repudiation of the procreative good of human sexuality, of marital intercourse, and of the human power to procreate.

It is certainly true that the need to abstain from marital relations in order to meet parental obligations and to avoid making oneself willing to reject an integral part of his or her personhood brings serious problems for married persons, which are poignantly illumined in those who have a serious obligation to prevent, as far as morally possible, the crippling of a child through a hereditary disease. But perhaps it would be better to say that this need brings them a cross, an opportunity to deepen their love for one another and for the God who gave them the great gift of sexuality, with its unitive and procreative dimensions, as a gift of their personhood. It gives them a chance to discover new ways of expressing their love for one another and for God.

Finally, it ought to be remembered that the conception and birth of a child who will be handicapped or perhaps even suffer as a result of a hereditary disease is *not* an unmitigated tragedy, an evil that is to be avoided at all costs. There is a serious moral responsibility to do what rightfully can be done to prevent the deterioration of the human genetic pool and avoid knowingly placing burdens on life-to-be-born, but we do not meet this responsibility by rejecting our humanity or by opting for the most efficient technical means for realizing its objectives.

Natural Family Planning, Spontaneous Abortion, and "Defective" Children

The famous German moral theologian, Bernard Häring, posits that "there is an undeniable relationship between the frequency of spontaneous abortion and the overripeness of spermatozoa and especially of the ova. Does this not mean that the rhythm method acts frequently rather as a means of 'birth control' and not simply as contraception, whenever it allows fertilization with aging gametes?"[26] Häring further contends that the "rhythm" method of contraception, inasmuch as it sometimes results in the fertilization of overripe gametic cells, leads to the birth of children who suffer from diseases induced by chromosomal disorders.[27]

It is instructive to note first that Häring insists on speaking of rhythm as a form of "contraception" and that he also seems to infer that rhythm is the only method of natural family planning. Since we have already shown that it is quite false to consider methods of family planning requiring periodic abstinence from marital intercourse as a "contraceptive" practice, there is no need here to linger further on this faulty basis of Häring's views. But it is necessary to take seriously his claim that rhythm is itself conducive to spontaneous abortions and to the incidence of children crippled by chromosomal diseases caused by the fertilization of aged germ cells.

In developing his thesis Häring relies principally on the investigations of R. V. Guerrero and O. I. Rojas.[28] In an exceptionally thorough study in which all of the pertinent scientific literature to date is taken into account, Dr. Thomas J. Hilgers has shown quite conclusively that the studies conducted on *animals* and on special populations of *humans* under unusual circumstances in no way leads to the conclusions reached by Häring with respect to the incidence of spontaneous abortions caused by the fertilization of aging gametic cells. Hilgers notes that there are many protective mechanisms that in nature prevent such a possibility from occurring; in particular, the fact that the cervical mucus of the human female acts like a biological valve. During certain times of the menstrual cycle, limited to the period shortly before and shortly after ovulation, the valve is open and sperm can penetrate and unite with the ovum to bring into being new life. At other times during the menstrual cycle this valve is closed and sperm cannot enter.[29]

Hilgers also shows that the statistics given by Häring and many other writers concerning enormous early embryological loss in humans must be seriously challenged. Häring and others rely primarily on work done by Drs. John Rock and A. T. Herting, involving the ova and embryonic life found in the wombs of women who received hysterectomies because of the pathological condition of their uteruses. It is quite obvious that any statistics concerning early embryonic loss or concerning abnormalities in embryos predicated upon studies carried out with this population of pregnant women can hardly be extended to prognosticate "normal wastage" in human pregnancies.[30]

Hilgers, toward the conclusion of his penetrating essay, comments on Häring's assertion that no competent scientist would find his own conclusions, namely, that "rhythm" is itself a cause of enormous embryonic wastage and chromosomally damaged children, in any way arbitrary or false. Hilgers simply says: "This is one scientist, actively involved in the research on and study of human reproduction, who feels that the hypotheses are arbitrary and the alarms false, while the reader can be assured that the author has exhaustively worked through the whole literature and all the arguments."[31]

Nor is Hilgers the only competent gynecologist who believes, after a careful study of the pertinent scientific data, that Häring is simply ignorant in reaching the conclusions he does. Dr. Josef Roetzer and Dr. Rudolf Vollmann both criticize severely the scientific methodology used by Guerrero (on whom Häring relies so heavily), terming it "statistical childish amusement with inhomogenous data and questionable methodology." They go on to say that the conclusions reached by Häring on the basis of these studies are simply an *"extrapolatio ad absurdum."*[32]

The perils Häring portrays concerning spontaneous abortions and "defective" children resulting from the exercise of parental responsibilities through periodic abstinence are in no way warranted. In addition, *even if* his position did have a scientific grounding, all it would mean would be that couples seeking to exercise their parental obligations through natural family planning methods would be required to forego intercourse for more days during each cycle in order to forestall fertilization of aging gametic cells.

It is not the purpose, in this concluding section of this chapter, to offer a full-length rebuttal to the argument advanced by Häring, but simply to call attention to the deficiencies in his argument as noted by competent members of the scientific community. There are ways for taking action that can help prevent the deterioration of the human genetic pool that are *not* morally objectionable. It is possible that the means suggested here may not be, in the short run, as efficient or economical in terms of human expenditure, as contraceptive intercourse, the sterilization of persons with recessive genetic defects, or the abortion of children suspected of being actually crippled by a hereditary disease. But in terms of what actions have to tell us about ourselves and our humanity, the means advocated here are more worthy of human endeavor, more responsive to the call to choose life and to communicate life and love to a future generation of human beings, that they are more conducive to fostering a covenant of grace among the productive generations of humankind.

Chapter 5

1. On this point see the illuminating discussion of human obligations in Charles Powers, John Simon, and Jon Gunnemann, *The Ethical Investor* (New Haven: Yale University Press, 1970).

2. On this see the discussion in chapter 3 above, pp. 00–00.

3. On this see Gerald Leach, *The Biocrats* (Baltimore: Penguin, 1972), pp. 139–153.

4. W. French Anderson, "Genetic Therapy," in Michael Hamilton, ed., *The New Genetics and the Future of Man* (Grand Rapids: Eerdmans, 1972), p. 109.

5. *Ibid.*, p. 117.

6. See Paul Ramsey's comments on Anderson's article in *op. cit.*, pp. 157–178. See also, Ramsey, "Morals and the Practice of Genetic Medicine," in *The Pilgrim People*, ed. Joseph Papin (Villanova, Pa.: Villanova University Press, 1973), pp. 71–84. See also the discussion in Charles Curran, *Politics, Medicine, and Ethics: A Dialogue With Paul Ramsey* (Philadelphia: Fortress, 1973), pp. 166–173.

7. Anderson, *loc. cit.*, p. 117.

8. *Ibid.*

9. Ramsey, *loc. cit.*

10. Leach, *op. cit.*, p. 157.

11. On this see Maureen Harris, ed., *Early Diagnosis of Human, Genetic Defects: Scientific and Ethical Considerations* (Fogarty International Center Proceedings, No. 6, 1972).

12. The best available source is John and Sheila Kippley, *The Art of Natural Family Planning* (Cincinnati: Couple to Couple League, 1975).

13. On this see Robert and Mary Joyce, *New Dynamics in Sexual Love* (Collegeville, Minn.: St. John's College Press, 1975).

14. See John and Sheila Kippley, *op. cit.*

15. See Bernard Häring, *Ethics of Manipulation* (New York: Seabury, 1975), pp. 92–96. Häring explicitly calls rhythm (which he seems to equate with all forms of natural family planning methods) a method of contraception.

16. James Burtchaell, " 'Human Life' and Human Love," originally published in *Commonweal*, Nov. 15, 1968, and reprinted in Paul Jersild and Dale Johnson, eds., *Moral Issues and Christian Response* (New York: Harper & Row, 1971), pp. 139–145.

17. In addition to the works referred to in the preceding notes see Michael Novak, "Frequent, Even Daily Communion," in Daniel Callahan, ed., *The Catholic Case for Contraception* (New York: Macmillan, 1969), pp. 92–102, esp. pp. 94–95.

18. On the difference between *meaning well* and *speaking well* through one's choices and actions see James O'Reilly, *The Moral Problem of Contraception* (Chicago: Franciscan Herald Press, 1975), p. 17. O'Reilly's booklet is one of the best short studies of contraception.

19. One of the clearest discussions of the differences between motives, intentionality, and consequences is Paul Ramsey's *The Just War* (New York: Scribner's, 1968), pp. 408–409.

20. On the importance of human acts as revelatory of our being see the Introduction and Herbert McCabe, *What Is Ethics All About?* (Washington: Corpus, 1969), pp. 92–101.

21. See *Summa Theologiae*, 1–2, 20, 1. See also chapter 4 of my *Becoming Human: An Invitation to Christian Ethics* (Dayton: Pflaum, 1975).

22. See McCabe, *op. cit.*, pp. 92–101.

23. A good history of this issue is given by John T. Noonan in his *Contraception* (Cambridge, Mass.: Harvard University Press, 1965). But Noonan's historical study needs to be supplemented by the works cited in the following footnote.

24. There is good reason for believing that St. Bonaventure and St. Thomas Aquinas, among others, began to realize that marital intercourse could be quite morally justifiable for goods other than procreation or, in a somewhat negative way, avoiding fornication. See the texts of these authors analyzed by Germain Grisez in "Marriage: Reflections on St. Thomas and Vatican II," *The Catholic Mind*, 64 (June 1966), and by Fabian Parmisano in "Love and Marriage in the Middle Ages I" and "Love and Marriage in the Middle Ages II," *New Blackfriars*, 50 (August and September 1969). These studies correct some interpretations of Noonan.

25. *Humanae Vitae*, par. 13.

26. Häring has set forth his views in two articles: "Genetics and Responsible Parenthood," *Social Thought,* 2 (Summer 1976): 7–14, and "New Dimensions of Responsible Parenthood," *Theological Studies,* 37 (March 1976): 120–132. The second essay is the most extensive presentation of his views.

27. That Häring has in mind chiefly the "rhythm" method is quite evident from his own words.

28. R. V. Guerrero, *Time of Insemination in the Menstrual Cycle and Its Effect on the Sex Ratio* (thesis, Harvard School of Public Health, 1968); R. V. Guerrero and O.I. Rojas, "Spontaneous Abortion and Aging Human Ova and Spermatozoa," *New England Journal of Medicine* 293:12 (September 18, 1975) 573–575.

29. Thomas J. Hilgers, M.D., "Human Reproduction: Three Issues for the Moral Theologian," *Theological Studies* 38.1 (March, 1977). pp. 136-52.

30. *Ibid.,* pp. 147–49.

31. *Ibid.,* pp. 150–51.

32. Josef Roetzer, M.D. and Rudolf Vollmann, cited in *Newsletter of the Human Life Center* 2.2 (June 1, 1976) 5.

6: Care of the Dying

The need to develop a sound moral policy of caring for the dying, along with the anguish and difficulty in doing so, was dramatically illustrated by the case of Karen Anne Quinlan of New Jersey, who was admitted to a hospital on April 15, 1975, in a comatose state, after having consumed alcohol and barbiturates. In the fall of that year her parents, who had become convinced that she would never regain consciousness and was being kept alive only by a respirator, petitioned Judge Robert Muir of the Morris County Superior Court to grant them permission, as her guardian, to remove her from the respirator so that they could, in the words of her father, "place her body and soul in the tender loving hands of the Lord." In November 1975 Judge Muir ruled that he could not grant this petition, and among the reasons he cited in support of his ruling was the judgment that "humanitarian motives cannot justify the taking of human life."[1]

In the spring of 1976 the Supreme Court of New Jersey overruled Judge Muir and gave Karen's parents permission to have her removed from the respirator. Since the staff of St. Clare's Hospital, where she was hospitalized, was opposed to this procedure, she was transferred to a nursing home and the respirator was disconnected. Much to everyone's surprise, she continued to live, breathing spontaneously, though capable of taking life-sustaining nourishment only through a nasal tube. At the time of this writing (December 1976), she still lives, and her parents and others still face the question of giving her the care she needs and that they are obligated to provide.

Since the "right-making or wrong-making features of medical care will not pop up from concentrating attention on a particular case,"[2] we will not try to derive them from the case of Karen Quinlan. Rather, by examining the moral issues that have come to the fore in the contemporary debate between the advocates of euthanasia and its opponents, we shall try to articulate the basic moral principles that can be of value in helping us give dying persons the kind of care they require. In the sequel, we can see how these principles relate to the Quinlan case. Thus I propose (1) to offer some preliminary clarifications, (2) to examine the ethics of euthanasia, (3) to provide an alternative to the ethics of euthanasia and to criticize its presuppositions, and (4) to offer some concluding reflections.

Preliminary Clarifications

The term "euthanasia" is derived from the combination of two Greek words meaning a good or a happy death. Originally it made no difference whether the death was natural or induced by human agency. Although this meaning of the term is still found in modern dictionaries, the meaning that has become prevalent in our culture is "an act or method of causing death painlessly so as to end suffering."[3] Today, in other words, "euthanasia" is synonymous with "mercy killing."

In the extensive literature that deals with the care of the dying we often encounter the expressions *active* (or positive or direct) euthanasia and *passive* (or negative or indirect) euthanasia. In ordinary speech, such as we find in newspapers, "active euthanasia" retains the connotation of "mercy killing" and designates the directly willed inducement of death for merciful reasons. "Passive euthanasia," on the other hand, is frequently understood to mean allowing oneself or another person to die when this person is terminally ill and there is no obligation to continue life-supporting (or, perhaps better, death-prolonging) means because there is no reasonable hope of recovery.[4] As we shall see when we investigate the ethics of euthanasia, many advocates of mercy killing adopt this terminology, inasmuch as most people readily admit that there are times when it is morally right, and indeed obligatory, to allow a dying person to die. Thus the advocates of the ethics of euthanasia or mercy killing argue that since passive euthanasia is widely accepted as a morally proper response to the needs of the dying, active euthanasia also should be a morally proper response in particular circumstances. I therefore suggest, with other writers, that we abandon this terminology and use "euthanasia" to refer to willingly inducing death, either by active means (administration of a lethal drug) or by "benign neglect," and a term such as "agathanasia" or "benemortasia" to refer to care of the dying that refuses to kill another human being, either by active means or neglect, for reasons of compassion. The reasons for this terminology will become clear as we proceed.

There are, as we shall see, very good reasons why we have the right, and even the obligation, to allow the dying to die their own death. But there is a world of difference between allowing or permitting death and deliberately setting out to bring death about. We ought not, it will be argued, deliberately seek death, either for ourselves or others. Human life, though by no means the absolute good or *summum bonum,* is nonetheless a real good of human beings. It is a good gift of the loving God of the covenant, for which we ought to have great love. Although we are not obliged to ward off death at all costs, we are obliged to love life and should not deliberately and of set purpose regard life as an evil or as a nongood.

Death, as such, is an evil. It is the privation of a good that is proper and fitting for the human person. It is not, of course, the greatest evil; it is the natural terminus of our life, something we can never escape. It is the meeting point of time and eternity. Each of us is to die and each of us is to learn to accept his or her death. But death, as such, is *not* a good. We ought, therefore, never directly will the death of a human person or wish to see anyone dead. We may, of course, wish to help a person face death and accept it humanly, but this is not the same as wanting a person to die or wishing to see a person dead.

With these clarifications we can begin our examination of the ethics of euthanasia.

The Ethics of Euthanasia

An increasing number of contemporary authors articulate the ethics of euthanasia. Although, as we shall see, there are significant differences among its proponents, all advocates of euthanasia or "mercy killing" (the term preferred by Daniel Maguire) [5] give an affirmative answer to the question "whether, in certain circumstances, we may intervene creatively to achieve death by choice." [6] All concur in holding that we can, as Joseph Fletcher puts it, "morally justify taking it into our own hands to hasten death for ourselves (suicide) or for others (mercy killing) ." [7] They all affirm that at times, as Maguire expresses it, it is "morally right and reasonable to terminate life through either positive action or calculated benign neglect." [8]

By examining the arguments of three representative proponents of the ethics of euthanasia we can discern the presuppositions that underlie the defense of this practice and then can contrast this ethics with an alternative approach to the care of the dying. The three proponents whose views we will examine are Joseph Fletcher, Marvin Kohl, and Daniel Maguire.

Joseph Fletcher, an Episcopalian clergyman (currently Visiting Professor of Medical Ethics at the Medical School of the University of Virginia) , has long been a champion of euthanasia. He holds that there are two basic forms or types of euthanasia, direct or positive and indirect or negative. The first consists of direct actions, or acts of commission, designed to terminate the life of an individual for humane reasons. The second consists in doing nothing to keep a person alive, although means are available for doing so. It consists, in other words, in acts of omission. [9]

Fletcher notes that some moralists "claim to see a moral difference between deciding to end a life by deliberately doing something and deciding to end a life by deliberately *not* doing something." [10] Such moralists endorse negative or indirect euthanasia and condemn positive or direct euthanasia. But, Fletcher says, this is morally evasive and disingenuous, inasmuch as "the end or purpose of both negative and positive euthanasia is exactly the same: to contrive or bring about the patient's death." [11] Hence, since there is a consensus that negative euthanasia is morally justifiable, it follows that positive euthanasia is likewise morally permissible.[12]

It must be noted immediately that those who oppose an ethics of euthanasia distinguish *sharply* between directly killing a person by taking lethal action against him and allowing or permitting a person to die his own death, and we will analyze this distinction more closely later. It would be a very serious error, however, to confuse this distinction with Fletcher's distinction between positive or direct and negative or indirect euthanasia. Positive *and* negative euthanasia, as described by Fletcher, are acts of "mercy killing"; both are intended to bring about the death of the patient; both are lethal actions directed against a person's life. Hence the consensus to which Fletcher refers in speaking about negative or indirect euthanasia is nonexistent. He erroneously thinks it exists because he has misunderstood the distinction between causing death and allowing a person to die.

However, Fletcher does not build his case for euthanasia on the moral equivalence of deciding to end a life by deliberately doing something and by deliberately *not* doing something. Rather, he builds his case by stressing (1) the right of moral man to control physical nature, (2) the primacy of the principle of proportionate good, and (3) the supremacy of such goods as personal integrity and dignity over the good of biological life.

With respect to the first point, Fletcher insists on the "right of spiritual beings to use intelligent control over physical nature rather than to submit beastlike to its blind workings."[13] He then likens the morality of euthanasia to that of contraception, for he writes: "Death control, like birth control, is a matter of human dignity. Without it persons become puppets."[14] Elsewhere, Fletcher elaborated on the right of persons to exercise dominion over physical nature, including bodily life and its processes:

> Physical nature—the body and its members, our organs and their functions—all of these *things* are a part of "what is over against us," and if we live by the rules and conditions set in physiology or another *it* we are not *thou.* . . . Freedom, knowledge, choice, responsibility— all these things of personal or moral stature are in us, not *out there*. Physical nature is what is over against us, out there. It represents the world of *its*.[15]

Put in this light, bodily, physical life pertains to an impersonal world of nature, of "its." Man—that is, personal, conscious, rational man—has the right to dispose of this physical, impersonal world in order to enhance such moral values as freedom, choice, responsibility.

In his writings on euthanasia and elsewhere, Fletcher stresses that it is the end that justifies the means. He does not mean that *any* end can justify *any* means; rather, he means that we may rightfully choose to do evil or to effect a disvalue if there is a sufficient reason or proportionate good that will be served by doing so: "The priority of the end is paired with the principle of 'proportionate good'; any disvalue in the means must be outweighed by the value gained in the end."[16] In some of his writings Fletcher determines the goodness of the end that can serve as a proportionate reason for effecting evil by a utilitarian calculus, that is, by simply counting the number of people who will be helped and those who will be hurt as a result of the action, and then doing the deed that will benefit most.[17] But in the context of his writings on euthanasia, the proportionate good that serves as the end, that justifies an act of killing either oneself or another, is the good of personal integrity or human dignity.[18]

Thus, for Fletcher, the third justifying element for euthanasia is the supremacy of such personal goods, that is, consciously experienceable goods, such as dignity and integrity. For him, these are the highest goods, incomparably superior to such impersonal and subhuman goods as physical life.[19]

Marvin Kohl's approach is similar to Fletcher's. He distinguishes between passive and active euthanasia, categories corresponding to Fletcher's positive and negative euthanasia, as two forms of bringing about a quick and painless death.[20]

Kohl does not develop the relevance of the principle of proportionate good to the issue of euthanasia, but he stresses the supremacy of the human value of dignity in moral issues and he associates the "right" of moral man to dispose of his own bodily life, in accordance with his own rational choices, with the concept of dignity. Kohl thus concurs with the other two presuppositions that underlie Fletcher's defense of euthanasia.

In his understanding of "dignity" Kohl recognizes the ambiguity in the term and acknowledges that many oppose euthanasia on the grounds that it violates personal dignity. He believes that these opponents understand dignity as "an intrinsic characteristic of humans," connoting "excellences that set human beings apart from other species."[21] He is ready to affirm that human beings possess this type of intrinsic dignity but he argues that it is irrelevant to the discussion of euthanasia. For him, the dignity that is crucial in understanding the significance of euthanasia is "extrinsic human dignity," which consists in "having reasonable control over the major and significant aspects of one's life."[22] This, for him, is the overriding moral concern in determining the morality of beneficent euthanasia. Killing oneself or another can be an act of kindness and legitimate self-determination; moral man has a right to do this because it is only on the basis of this right that a human being will be guaranteed the dignity that is central to a self-determining being, namely, the dignity that denotes "the actual ability of a human being to rationally determine and control his way of life and death and to have this acknowledged and respected by others."[23] Thus it is evident that Kohl shares Fletcher's conviction that human dignity consists in man's rational control over his own life and that this kind of dignity functions as an absolute, as the "highest good" in moral choices.

Daniel Maguire, a Roman Catholic moralist, while differing from both Fletcher and Kohl in many significant ways,[24] concurs with them in affirming the moral right to choose death either for oneself (suicide) or for another (mercy killing) in specific circumstances; and the argument he develops to support this conclusion bears striking affinities to the argument developed by these other writers.

First, however, we should note a difference between Maguire and Fletcher. As we have seen, Fletcher misunderstands the distinction between deliberately intending to cause a person's death by lethal action and allowing or permitting a person to die his own death. Maguire understands the nature of this distinction and recognizes that it is morally valid and important. It is a valid distinction inasmuch as "to *will* an evil effect (death) is not the same as *permitting* the evil effect," and it is an important distinction inasmuch as "the moral quality of an act will be affected by the attitude of the will toward the evil effect."[25] Clearly, Maguire recognizes the meaning of this distinction and its moral significance, and in doing so sets himself somewhat apart from Fletcher.

But it would be a serious error to conclude that there is a great deal of difference between Maguire and Fletcher or Kohl in their approaches to euthanasia. Maguire's acceptance of the validity and significance of the distinction between killing a person by lethal action and allowing him to die can be explained by his background as a moralist who was educated in the Roman Catholic tradition, in which this distinction has a crucial role.[26]

What is most important to recognize is that Maguire, in company with a number of other Roman Catholic moral theologians, has concluded that this distinction plays only a very limited and subsidiary role in making good moral choices in conflict situations—that is, when, no matter what is done, some evil will come about. For Maguire and such writers as Cornelius Van der Poel,[27] William Van der Marck,[28] and Richard McCormick (who has articulated the position in most detail),[29] "more important than directness or indirectness is the question of whether there is a proportionate reason to permit or intend [an evil such as death]."[30]

This means that one can rightfully choose to do a deed that directly causes evil that the agent cannot not intend or will so long as there is a "proportionate reason." A greater proportionate reason may be required if one is rightfully to intend the evil directly than if one permits or allows the evil to occur,[31] but the "basic category" for determining whether the deed is morally permissible is proportionate reason.[32]

Applying this principle to suicide and mercy killing, Maguire holds that one can rightfully choose to kill himself or another if, by doing so, he protects or secures some good that is greater than that of physical life, such as personal integrity or the freedom of self-determination. In other words, there is a weighing of values or goods, and the good of physical life is judged of lesser value than that of personal integrity or dignity. Hence the choice to destroy life of set purpose can be a morally good choice, justified by the principle of proportionate reason.[33]

It is evident that Maguire's defense of suicide and mercy killing parallels that of Fletcher, for, like him, Maguire stresses the primacy, indeed the sufficiency, of the principle of proportionate reason and the supremacy of such goods as personal integrity and dignity over the "merely biological" good of life.[34]

Maguire also agrees with Fletcher in emphasizing the right that man—the conscious, rational subject—has to subject physical nature to his mastery, and in the world of physical nature Maguire includes bodily life, or what he terms "biochemical and organic factors." Thus he echoes Fletcher in comparing mercy killing to birth control. Just as birth control "was impeded by the physicalist ethic that left moral man at the mercy of his biology" until "technological man discover [ed] that he was morally free to intervene creatively and to achieve birth control by choice," the same physicalist ethic has long condemned him "to await the good pleasure of biochemical and organic factors and allow these to determine the time and the manner of his demise." But now, Maguire's argument runs, technological man can creatively intervene, and has a moral right to do so, "to terminate life through either positive action or calculated benign neglect rather than to await in awe the dispositions of organic tissue."[35]

From this survey of the arguments of three leading advocates of the ethics of euthanasia we see that they justify suicide and mercy killing when these acts are (a) well motivated, (b) protect or enhance the goods of personal integrity and dignity, which serve as proportionate reasons for intending an evil (death), and (c) are an expression of the dominion that rational and conscious beings (men) have over the physical world of nature, which includes their bodies and bodily life. It is also apparent that the advocates of beneficent euthanasia are consequentialistic in their moral reasoning; that is, they believe that the final determinants of the rightness or wrongness of our actions and practices are the consequences they bring about. They hold that the end justifies the means and that the ultimate, master rubric in moral questions is the principle of the proportionate good or reason.[36] The ethics of euthanasia, in short, can be termed an "ethics of intent" in which the ultimate determinant of the rightness or wrongness of what one does is the good or evil that is both intended by the agent and results from the action he undertakes.

The Ethics of Agathanasia or Benemortasia

The ethics of euthanasia, though motivated by compassion for those who are painfully and terminally ill and by respect for the basic human goods of dignity and freedom of choice, must be rejected as a way of providing for the dying the care they need·and that society is obligated to provide. It is, in my judgment, incompatible with a Christian understanding of human existence and the significance of human acts.

In what follows I will offer a critique of the ethics of euthanasia and then outline the ethics of "agathanasia" or "benemortasia." These terms were coined by the Protestant ethicists Paul Ramsey[37] and Arthur Dyck,[38] respectively, to stress the very real difference in the care of the dying as indicated by an ethics rooted in the Christian faith (and in a long tradition of Roman Catholic moral theology), as distinguished from the kind of care advocated by the champions of beneficent euthanasia or death by choice.

Critique of the Ethics of Euthanasia

Of the many serious objections that can be brought against the ethics of euthanasia, the following are the most important.

First, the ethics of euthanasia is a consequentialistic ethics, according absolute priority to the principle of proportionate reason or good and holding that one may rightfully intend evil so that good may come about. As we shall see, a proportionate reason or good is needed to justify doing deeds that effect evil, but the proportionate good that serves as the end to be achieved does not suffice to render deeds good and right. If we take the significane of our deeds seriously, as revelatory of our being and as shaping our identity, we must conclude that if we directly will or intend an evil, such as death, we show that we are willing to take on as part of our moral identity the identity of evildoers, for *evil is what we do* if it is an evil that cannot not be intended. We may do this evil reluctantly, and be tempted to *redescribe* our act of killing, whether this be suicide or mercy killing, in terms of the intended results by saying that what we are doing is "showing compassion" or "preserving human dignity."[39] But if the evil that is brought about by our deeds is an evil we directly intend or will, the acts in question are acts of killing, and no redescription can conceal this reality.

Also, if we look upon the significance of our deeds from a Christian perspective, mindful of being living images or created words of a loving God, we realize that we ought to be his faithful images and truthful words. And God is absolutely innocent of evil. He *permits* evil but does not set his will on it; he does not directly will or intend it to be.[40] If we are to be his faithful images, true to the Word he has given us in Jesus, we ought not be willing to choose to do a deed that of necessity requires us to intend the evil effected, for if we do we cannot be innocent of that evil. Rather, we are responsible for it.

Second, the ethics of euthanasia involves the weighing or "commensurating" of human goods and choosing some, for instance dignity or personal integrity, and rejecting or repudiating others, namely life itself. But no created human good is the *summum bonum,* the absolute good, and no created human good is an evil. Those who justify suicide and mercy killing claim that we can rightfully choose death—an evil that is privative of the good of life—for the sake of the "higher" or "greater" good of dignity or integrity. They thus maintain that life as such is not a good that is worthy of human choice[41] and they erect the goods of dignity and personal integrity into absolute goods, that is, goods whose protection and preservation is so important that they can justify our repudiation of other basic human goods.

This contention of the ethics of euthanasia is untenable. The various real goods that together make up the whole human good are all real goods of human beings, created participations in the goodness of God himself, who alone is the supreme good or *summum bonum.* Because they are all real goods, they merit our love and respect; each of these real good human goods, including life itself, is worthy of human choice. A sound moral policy, reflecting a heart that is open to all that is good and worthwhile, requires us to love and respect all the real goods of human beings, of human persons. These goods are not comparable and cannot be weighed one against another. To measure the good of dignity or of personal integrity against the good of life itself is like measuring the smile on a child's face against the thrill of Newton in discovering the laws of gravity. It's comparing the incomparable, weighing the unweighable. It is, in other words, an exercise in folly.[42]

Third, the ethics of euthanasia, as articulated by Fletcher and Maguire, betrays a false understanding of the human person. For them, man is not an indissoluble union of body and soul, he is the Cartesian ghost in a machine, for they regard man's humanity as exhausted by his consciousness and rationality and his body and biological life as a subpersonal, subhuman component, part of a "world of nature" over which the rational and conscious agent has complete dominion. This view of man is incompatible with the biblical and Christian understanding of the human person as a special kind of animal, as the "body of his soul" and the "soul of his body."[43]

The ethics of euthanasia is indeed, as Arthur Dyck has shown so clearly, not new but is a contemporary articulation of Stoic philosophy.[44] It is admirable in many ways, for it values the true human goods of compassion, mercy, freedom, and integrity; but it does not do full justice to the meaning of human existence and to the range of human values.

Agathanasia/Benemortasia and Care of the Dying

A policy for providing proper care to the dying, I believe, is rooted in the ethics of agathanasia or benemortasia. With the advocates of euthanasia, we who propose the ethics of agathanasia/benemortasia agree that compassion, mercy, freedom, and dignity are human values. But the means we use to achieve these values, the deeds we choose to do to realize them, are equally important, for they tell us about the meaning of our lives as moral beings. The ethics of agathanasia/benemortasia is as concerned with means as it is with ends; it is not simply an ethics of intent but an *ethics of intent and content*. It does not regard the good consequences intended by an agent (the proportionate reason or good to be attained) as the principal determinant of the morality of the deeds or actions he chooses for attaining his ends. The meaning or significance of the deeds whereby he achieves his good purposes is equally a determinant of their morality. For an ethics of agathanasia/benemortasia, a human deed not only gets something *done,* that is, has consequences or results, but also gets something *said,* that is, it tells us about the meaning of our lives.[45] This ethics, consequently, recognizes that human freedom and dignity are not the absolutes into which they have been raised by the advocates of beneficent euthanasia. It recognizes that these values have certain constraints that enable human beings to be *humanly* free and *humanly* dignifed.

One of the constraints on human freedom and dignity and on enabling human beings to exercise compassion and freedom humanly is the constraint articulated in the commandment, "Thou shalt not kill." "The injunction not to kill," Professor Dyck writes,

> is part of a total effort to prevent the destruction of the human community. It is an absolute prohibition in the sense that no society can be indifferent about the taking of human life. Any act, *insofar as it is an act of taking a human life* [this is precisely what euthanasia, as an activity directly targeted on the destruction of human life by lethal attack, whether by positive act or benign neglect, is] is wrong; that is to say, that taking a human life is a wrong-making characteristic of actions. To say, however, that killing is a *prima facie* wrong does not mean that an act of killing [I would prefer to say "an act that results in death"] may never be justified. For example, a person's efforts to prevent someone's death may lead to the death of the attacker. However, we can morally justify that act of intervention only because it is an act of saving a life, not because it is an act of taking a life.[46]

We could put it this way. A human being ought not *directly and of deliberate intent* take human life, either his own or another's. We ought not do this, first of all, because life itself is a real human good, a created participation in the goodness of God himself, and as a result is a reality we ought to cherish and respect, rather than despise. Second, we ought not take a human life because no human being exists apart from other human beings; not only is human existence a co-existence, it is also a for-existence; not only is being human a being *with,* it is also a being *for.* We human beings exist *with* and *for* one another; each of us holds his life at the mercy of his fellows. Profound Christian meaning is at stake here, for we believe that human beings are the living images or icons of God. Just as the living and loving God is an Emmanuel, a God who exists as Karl Barth has noted, "neither *next* to man nor *above* him, but *with* him, *by* him, and above all *for* him"[47]—we, his images, are to exist with and for one another. This God is no killer of life; hence neither are we, his images and children, to be killers.

The ethics of agathanasia/benemortasia, however, is as opposed to vitalism and a "save and care" ethics, as described by Gerald Leach,[48] as is the ethics of euthanasia. In other words, agathanasia/ benemortasia holds that life itself is not the absolute good, the be-all and end-all of human existence, the *summum bonum.* Vitalists, such as Dr. David A. Karnofsky, erect life into the highest good and speak of the medical imperative to use every stratagem known to medicine to ward off death "until the issue is taken out of [the physician's] hands."[49] The euthanasists, on the other hand, erect the goods of human dignity and integrity into absolutes. The ethics of agathanasia/benemortasia values all human goods, including those of life, freedom, and integrity, but it recognizes that God alone is the *summum bonum,* the highest good, *the* absolute, and that man's *moral* good is constituted by his willingness to love all true goods of human beings as they ought to be loved and to love God above all created goods. Created human goods such as life and freedom are indeed to be loved and ought never to be repudiated or despised, but they are not to be loved as the be-all and end-all of human existence.

Thus human life is not a good that is to be clung to no matter what. If clinging to it, and attempting to preserve it, require us to *turn against* other human goods, such as dignity or freedom or integrity, such actions that preserve life are wrong, immoral. Although death is *not* a good and is *not* worthy of human choice— which is contrary to the claim of advocates of beneficent euthanasia—neither is it an evil that is to be prevented at all costs. It is an event that closes our mortal existence, a reality we must accept and experience and can never avoid. It is for this reason that a human being has the right to refuse medical interventions that needlessly prolong the dying process and prevent him from dying his own death and from accepting, in a humanly free and dignified way, the end of his mortal existence.

This is why the ethics of agathanasia/benemortasia maintains that we are not only morally free to allow or permit either others or ourselves to die but that at times we are morally obliged to do so. This ethics does take seriously the distinction between taking a life by lethal action, either by commission or omission, and permitting a person to die. It holds that we are morally obliged *not to kill* other human beings by direct intent, either by positive action or by failing to do what we reasonably can to prevent death (the "benign neglect" to which Maguire refers) when it is morally obligatory to do so. But it holds that we can, for sufficient reasons, *allow* a person to die. To see precisely what this means, let us look at the distinction between killing a person and letting a person die.

If we reflect on the human significance or meaning of our deeds we see that this distinction is valid. It is evident that human choice and human action are involved in both types of activity, but there is a vast moral difference in the way these actions are related to the moral identity of the responsible agents, in the way the deeds shape or form the agents' moral being. In actions that kill persons by commission (shooting them, giving them a lethal poison) or omission (failing to throw a life preserver to a drowning person if one can) the purpose or intent of both the act and the doer is to bring about death, to kill. Such actions may have different *motives,* but motives are not morally decisive in determining the meaning of actions. Whether I kill a person by shooting him or by failing to give him the food he needs in order to live, either because I despise him or feel compassion for him, I kill him, and have chosen to do a deed of killing. If, however, I choose to let a person die by not taking measures that could prolong his dying process, I have not chosen to kill him, either by an act of commission or an act of omission. As Dr. J. Russell Elkinton noted, "It is morally decisive that the patient dies not from the act but from the underlying disease or injury."[50] Dr. C. B. Giertz puts it this way: "No step is taken with the object [intent] of killing the patient. We refrain from treatment because it does not serve any purpose. . . . I cannot regard this as killing by medical means: death has already won, despite the fight we have put up."[51]

More positively, we can say, with Ramsey, that the decision not to administer life-sustaining (better, death-postponing) technologies or to cease employing them is a choice to *care* for the dying person, to minister to his needs as a human being in the process of dying, and to make his dying an act at which human presence and human concern are of greater value than tubes inserted into his nose, rectum, or other openings.[52]

We can morally and, indeed, *ought* morally to allow human beings to die their own death; but there must be a sufficient or proportionate reason for making this choice. The principle of sufficient or proportionate reason (or good) is relevant to the care of the dying, but it is not the "master category" in ethics. Associated with this principle is the principle of intentionality, which means that in choosing to allow a person to die we do not set our will against his life by intending to kill him. When *both* criteria are met, when both of these valid moral principles are operative, we can rightfully choose to allow a person to die and to care for that person in his act of dying.

The great difficulty is in determining whether there are sufficient reasons, a proportionate good, for allowing death to happen. Traditionally, medical ethics has distinguished between *ordinary* and *extraordinary* means of preserving life, the former have been regarded as mandatory or obligatory, and to omit them is the moral equivalent of killing a patient (terminating his life by Maguire's benign neglect), whereas the latter have been regarded as elective.[53] The distinction between ordinary and extraordinary means or mandatory and elective procedures must not be misunderstood, as many moralists, as well as Pope Pius XII, have noted repeatedly.[54] It is not a "facile" distinction, as Maguire asserts in one of his articles,[55] nor is it a gimmick to save consciences. It is a difficult distinction to make but one that good medicine can and must make.

The terms "ordinary" and "extraordinary" are to be taken in their moral sense, which need not coincide with their meaning in a *technological* sense. A procedure that may be ordinary in the medically technological sense (e.g., intravenous feeding, a heart pacemaker, etc.), because it is commonly followed and readily available, may be extraordinary in the moral sense. The terms have great relativity, not because of any moral relativism, but because they are *relative to the condition of the patient,* to the morally significant reality-making and truth-making factors that give them their moral meaning. Intravenous feeding or an operation that is ordinary and mandatory for a patient of a certain age, with a particular kind of disease or injury and reasonable hope of recovery, might be extraordinary and might constitute a senseless and brutal prolongation of the dying process and hence be directed against the integrity and dignity of a 95-year-old person in a coma, suffering from bone cancer, renal failure, and pneumonia. Among the factors that are reality-making in determining the condition of the patient are his freedom to die the death he is in fact dying and the fact that he has already begun the process of dying. Although it is no easy task to determine the condition of the patient, and human errors can be made in determining it, this task is at the heart of the care that physicians and medical science must extend to dying human beings.

Richard McCormick S.J., believes that we must go beyond the "extraordinary-ordinary means" distinction to make *quality-of-life* judgments in determining the care we are to give dying persons. It will be useful to examine his proposals, for by reflecting on them we will be able to understand more clearly the distinction between ordinary and extraordinary means as an aid in determining when there are sufficient reasons for allowing a person to die.

McCormick believes that in determining whether a medical procedure constitutes ordinary or extraordinary means we must arrange the various components of the total human good into a hierarchy and that "in the Judeo-Christian perspective, the meaning, substance, and consummation of life are found in human *relationships,* and the qualities of justice, respect, concern, compassion and support that surround them."[56] Life, in the sense of physical or biological life, is indeed one of the components of the human good. It is "basic and precious," but it is, he says, "a good to be preserved precisely as the condition of other values."[57] In the sense of physical or biological life, life "is a value to be preserved only insofar as it contains some potentiality for human relationships."[58]

When I first read McCormick's reflections I interpreted them to mean that life itself, in the sense of physical or biological life, is simply what an older terminology would have termed a *bonum utile* or useful good, not a *bonum honestum* or intrinsic good, whereas such relational human goods as justice and friendship and compassion are *bona honesta* and hence "higher" or "greater" goods.[59] But if we reread the passage carefully, we see that this may be only partially true. It is definitely true, for McCormick, that such relational goods as justice and friendship are "higher" goods than physical life, but perhaps he does not regard life itself simply as a useful good or *bonum utile*. He recognizes that it is "basic and precious," and his point seems to be that there is *no obligation* to preserve the good of physical life when there is no possibility that the relational and higher goods can be achieved. I believe this is the way his comments ought to be interpreted.

McCormick then proposes that a medical means is extraordinary, and hence not mandatory, when there is no longer any potentiality for human relationships.[60] When this is the case, it follows from his argument that there is no longer any obligation to preserve life and that one can rightfully let a person die.

Although this is apparently the way McCormick intends his comments to be understood, I worry about them. Even though he seems to recognize that physical life is inherently good (a *bonum honestum*), he seems to locate its goodness in its *function* as a basis for other, "higher" goods. Thus it is very hard to see how it can be a good in any sense when this function that it performs ceases. It would seem to be a *non*good.

Also, we must be very careful in speaking about the "hierarchy" of human goods. There is a sense in which friendship is a higher good than life, and a friend will willingly sacrifice his life for the good of a friend—he will die rather than betray his friendship—but this does not mean that his life is no longer a good that he must love and respect. He can never despise his life or set his will (his intent) against it, for it remains a good gift from

God, a true component of the human good. In truth, the components of the human good are incommensurable. We cannot compare them with one another, weigh one against the other, and choose against one in preference for another. To compare life itself with friendship or compassion or justice is like comparing a sunset to a child's smile or the thrill of Archimedes when he exclaimed *"Eureka!"* These realities are incomparable, immeasurable.

Yet the weighing of values is precisely what McCormick advocates in his general moral theory, for he is the foremost exponent of the ethics of the proportionate good. He is the leader in affirming that the principle of the proportionate good is the "master category"[61] in the ethics that is reflected in Maguire's defense of mercy killing and suicide. Again, in his essay on saving or letting die McCormick concluded that medical means are extraordinary and that it is therefore permissible *not* to preserve life and to let a person die when the potentiality of biological life for the "higher" goods of human relationships has been exhausted. Although he did not conclude that it would then be morally permissible to destroy life by deliberate intent, this conclusion is contained in his premises—and it is this conclusion that Maguire drew in his defense of our right to "choose death" and to "terminate," that is, destroy, life "through either positive action or calculated benign neglect." In fact, Maguire points out that McCormick's only objections to his "death-by-choice" ethics are predicated on consequentialistic grounds. McCormick worries whether in the long run the effect of this ethics on the good of life will be detrimental.[62]

I therefore believe that McCormick's proposal for making quality-of-life judgments in order to determine whether a medical procedure constitutes ordinary or extraordinary means must be rejected. Still, his proposal illumines the problem. Qualities such as justice, friendship, concern, and the like *are* components of the whole human good, along with life itself. As true human goods they merit our love and respect, and it would be wrong to engage in acts that are directly destructive of them, just as it is wrong, deliberately and of set purpose, to engage in acts that are directly destructive of the good of life. Consequently, if medical interventions that could, in one sense, preserve life (though I believe it would be better to describe them as prolonging the dying process) are foreseen to hinder the dying person's participation in these human goods, they constitute extraordinary means and are no longer morally obligatory. In fact, if their use or continued use not only hinders the dying person's participation in these human goods but positively destroys them in that person, there is a moral obligation to refrain from or to discontinue their use inasmuch as the choice to use them is the equivalent of destroying these human goods in a dying person.

To summarize the ethics of agathanasia/benemortasia it will be helpful, I believe, to articulate its presuppositions. They have been well stated by Arthur Dyck[63] and can be summarized as follows:

1. A human being's life is not solely at the disposal of that person; every human life is part of a human community that is held together, in part, by respect for life and love for the lives of its members.
2. The dignity of the person, by reason of his freedom of choice, includes the freedom of dying persons to refuse non-curative, death-preventing interventions, but it does not include the freedom to choose death and to set one's will against life.
3. Every life has worth. Life itself is a precious good; it is a *bonum honestum* or intrinsic good and not a *bonum utile* or merely conditional good.
4. The supreme good is God himself, to whom the dying and those who care for the dying are responsible.

Concluding Reflections and the Karen Quinlan Case

To care properly for the dying is one of the greatest challenges confronting contemporary society, which, as noted earlier, was dramatically presented to the American public by the Karen Quinlan case. Karen still lives, but in my judgment there is no moral obligation, by the ethics of agathanasia/benemortasia, to use the means that are currently employed to prolong her death. Morally, her parents, and others, could remove the tubes that are necessary for her feeding, prevent dehydration by appropriate medical means, and attend to her in her dying moments.

But Karen Quinlan is *not,* as some have maintained in commenting on the case, a "vegetable." She is a living human being, a being of moral worth. With Thomas C. Oden, I believe there is a very dangerous tendency, which needs to be resisted with all possible vigor, to consider persons in her condition as no more than "living vegetables." Calling such persons by this term "amounts to a linguistic predisposition and rationale to act as if the patient were a vegetable. It provides a convenient language for the predisposition of crucial moral decisions. It is a pejorative, prejudicial, and dehumanizing use of metaphor."[64]

Although Judge Muir, in ruling that Karen's parents could not be authorized, as her guardians, to remove her from the respirator, may have made a mistake, I believe his decision is evidence of greater moral sensitivity than the decision of the Supreme Court of New Jersey, which overruled him. The case before Judge Muir was ineptly argued, in the judgment of many,[65] but he was surely correct in resisting the beneficent euthanasia rationale that was developed by many in their eagerness to have the respirator turned off so that a "vegetable" would cease to exist. Muir did not, I believe, give sufficiently serious attention to the distinction between extraordinary and ordinary means,[66] but in holding that "humanitarian motives cannot justify the taking of a human life" he expressed a basic presupposition of the ethics of agathanasia/benemortasia, as against the ethics of euthanasia.

The Supreme Court of New Jersey's ruling was hailed by some as "just great,"[67] but I believe there is cause for concern over its ruling. Part of its decision is as follows:

> We believe, first, that the ensuing death would not be homicide but rather expiration from existing natural causes. [I and those who advocate the ethics of agathanasia/benemortasia agree.] Secondly, *even if it were to be regarded as homicide, it would not be unlawful. . . . There is a real and in this case determinative distinction between the unlawful taking of the life of another and the ending of artificial life-support systems as a matter of self-determination.*[68] [Emphasis added.]

I believe that the Supreme Court of New Jersey's ruling is a legalization of the ethics of euthanasia, or at least a step in that direction. The court put great stress on the values of consciousness, cognitiveness, and sapientness. Too many in our society are eager to confer beneficent euthanasia on dying persons who lack these qualities. Thus to establish them as absolutely determinative is a serious error.[69]

I believe that Oden provides useful guidelines for persons who face the responsibility of caring for the dying and whose conscience comes into conflict with that of attending physicians, who might (almost subconsciously) be overly influenced by the technological imperative to do everything until the matter is completely taken out of their hands. Oden writes:

> Where there is a conflict of conscience between the conscience of the physician and the conscience of the family, pastoral care should intervene to help the family negotiate, at an early stage, a change of doctors, or if that fails, a change of hospitals. For different physicians and different hospitals have different interpretations of standard medical practice and "extraordinary treatment."
>
> If the above measures fail, pastoral care will assist the family in a careful examination of conscience. If they are perfectly clear in conscience that the patient should be allowed to die without further medical interventions, they may begin a carefully paced sequence of withholding consent on several levels, with time allowed between each level: first, to withhold consent to treatment of new infections; second, if necessary, to respiration; third, only if necessary, from other forms of emergency or intensive care; and finally, only if necessary, from all forms of treatment, including high-caloric intravenous feeding. If all these measures have failed, they can withhold consent from hospitalization itself, but this should be done only after all reasonable efforts have been made to transfer the patient to another hospital.[70]

Chapter 6

1. The citations from Karen Quinlan's father and from Judge Muir's decision are taken from articles in "The Quinlan Decision," *Hastings Center Report,* 6 (February 1976): 8–19.

2. Paul Ramsey, "Prolonged Dying: Not Medically Indicated," in *ibid.,* p. 14.

3. *New World Dictionary,* College Edition (New York: World, 1962), under entry "euthanasia."

4. On this see Kevin D. O'Rourke O.P., "Active and Passive Euthanasia: The Ethical Distinctions," *Hospital Progress* (November 1976), p. 68.

5. Daniel Maguire, "A Catholic View of Mercy Killing," in *Beneficent Euthanasia,* ed. Marvin Kohl (Buffalo: Prometheus, 1975), p. 42, n. 6.

6. Daniel Maguire, "The Freedom to Die," in *New Theology No. 10,* ed. Martin Marty and Dean Peerman (New York: Macmillan, 1973), p. 188.

7. Joseph Fletcher, "Ethics and Euthanasia," *American Journal of Nursing,* 73 (April 1973): 673. This essay was later printed as a chapter in *To Live and To Die,* ed. Robert H. Williams (New York: Springer Verlag, 1973).

8. Maguire, "The Freedom to Die," p. 189.

9. Fletcher develops this distinction of the two forms of euthanasia in "Ethics and Euthanasia," *loc. cit.,* and in his essay "The Patient's Right to Die," in *Euthanasia and the Right to Death,* ed. A. B. Downing (London: Peter Owen, 1969), pp. 66–69.

10. Fletcher, "The Patient's Right to Die," p. 68.

11. Fletcher, "Ethics and Euthanasia," p. 675.

12. *Ibid.,* pp. 670–671.

13. Fletcher, "The Patient's Right to Die," p. 69.

14. *Ibid.*

15. Joseph Fletcher, *Morals and Medicine* (Boston: Beacon, 1960), p. 211.

16. Fletcher, "Ethics and Euthanasia," p. 674.

17. See, e.g., his *Situation Ethics* (Philadelphia: Westminster, 1965).

18. This is clearly brought out in both "Ethics and Euthanasia" and "The Patient's Right to Die." See also Fletcher's more recent essay, "The 'Right' to Live and the 'Right' to Die," in *Beneficent Euthanasia,* pp. 44–56.

19. See, e.g., "Ethics and Euthanasia," p. 674.

20. Marvin Kohl, "Voluntary Beneficent Euthanasia," in *Beneficent Euthanasia,* p. 131.

21. *Ibid.,* pp. 132–133.

22. *Ibid.*, p. 133.

23. *Ibid.*

24. Maguire is by no means the calculating utilitarian that Fletcher, in most of his writings, is. Unlike Fletcher, Maguire is not, at bottom, a noncognitivist in ethical theory for he believes that we can get to know the truth about our selves and our acts and that moral judgments are not only capable of being "validated" but of being verified or falsified, that is, of being shown to be true or false. Still, Maguire is, like Fletcher, a consequentialist, as will become evident as we proceed.

It should be noted that Maguire frequently, in his writings on death by choice, appeals to the teaching of St. Thomas about the applicability of moral principles in particular cases. He appeals particularly to the teaching of St. Thomas in *Summa Theologiae,* 1–2, 94, aa. 4 and 5, that moral norms are valid only *in pluribus,* that is, in most of the cases. Thomas, in the context referred to, refers to a principle to return something that someone has borrowed to its rightful owner and to the fact that at times, because the owner is mad or for some other reason, there is no longer a moral obligation to do so. There is no opportunity here to go into the exegesis of St. Thomas, but it can be said that Maguire completely misinterprets him. St. Thomas definitely held that some actions are inherently or intrinsically evil and that such actions cannot rightfully be done, despite the consequences. He held that some moral rules are really exceptionless, not merely virtually so.

For an excellent discussion of the Thomistic texts in question see R. A. Armstrong, *Primary and Secondary Precepts in Thomistic Natural Law Teaching* (The Hague: Martinus Nijhoff, 1966). Armstrong's careful study, along with such superb commentaries on Thomas's moral theory as Germain Grisez's "The Primary Principle of the Natural Law: A Commentary on the *Summa Theologiae,* 1–2, 94, 2," *Natural Law Forum,* 10 (1965): 168–196, will enable the reader to appreciate the misuse to which the Thomistic texts, cited by Maguire in his various writings on mercy killing, have been put.

25. Daniel Maguire, *Death by Choice* (New York: Doubleday, 1974), p. 120.

26. For the importance of this distinction and its relationship to the rule or principle of double effect see Germain G. Grisez, "Toward a Consistent Natural-Law Ethics of Killing," *American Journal of Jurisprudence,* 15 (1970): 64–96; Joseph Mangan, "An Historical Analysis of the Principle of Double Effect," *Theological Studies,* 10 (1949): 41–61; and my article "Double Effect, Principle of," in *Encyclopedia of Bioethics,* ed. Warren Reich (New York: Macmillan, 1978).

27. Cornelius Van der Poel, *The Search for Human Values* (New York: Newman, 1971).

28. William Van der Marck, *Toward a Christian Ethic* (New York: Newman, 1967).

29. Richard McCormick, *Ambiguity in Moral Choice* (Milwaukee: Marquette University Press, 1973). McCormick has developed this ethics of the proportionate good in his "Notes in Moral Theology" in *Theological Studies* and sees it as the converging point toward which contemporary Roman Catholic moral theologians are working. It is an ethics that is vigorously opposed by such writers as Germain Grisez and Paul Ramsey, who will soon publish extensive critiques of it. I have offered criticisms of this development in contemporary Roman Catholic moral theology in my book *Becoming Human: An Invitation to Christian Ethics* (Dayton: Pflaum, 1975) and in my article "Ethics and Human Identity: The Challenge of the New Biology," *Horizons: The Journal of the College Theology Society*, 3 (1976): 17–37.

30. Maguire, "A Catholic View of Mercy Killing," pp. 39–40. He correctly goes on to say that the importance given to the principle of proportionate reason "opens the way to a revolution in Catholic thinking in areas such as mercy killing." It most certainly does, for it amounts to a repudiation of the entire Roman Catholic tradition.

31. McCormick brings this out in his *Ambiguity in Moral Choice*.

32. McCormick terms the principle of proportionate reason or good the "basic category" in *Ambiguity*, p. 77. Maguire accepts it as such, as the master rubric in "doing" ethics, in his *Death by Choice*, pp. 126–128.

33. This is the basic argument developed by Maguire in *Death by Choice*, "The Freedom to Die," and "A Catholic View of Mercy Killing."

34. Maguire most clearly brings out his belief that the goods of personal, conscious existence far outweigh the good of merely "biological life" in his "Freedom to Die" essay.

35. *Ibid.*, pp. 188–189.

36. Fletcher translates the supremacy of proportionate good into the formula "the end justifies the means." Maguire does not use this language, but McCormick, from whom he draws much of his inspiration, puts it into Latin, for he says that we may rightfully intend evil *in se* but not *propter se* or that we may rightfully intend evil *in se in ordine ad finem proportionatum.* See his "Notes in Moral Theology," *Theological Studies*, 33 (1972): 74–75. As I understand Latin, this is the equivalent of the English expression "The end justifies the means."

37. Ramsey coins the word in his long essay "On (Only) Caring for

the Dying" in his *Patient as Person* (New Haven: Yale University Press, 1970), pp. 113–164. The term "agathanasia" is from two Greek words meaning literally a "good" "death".

38. Arthur Dyck develops the notion of benemortasia in two places: "An Alternative to an Ethics of Euthanasia," in *To Live and To Die,* pp. 98–112, and in "Beneficent Euthanasia and Benemortasia: Alternative Views of Mercy," in Kohl's anthology, *Beneficent Euthanasia,* pp. 117–129. The term "benemortasia" is from two Latin words meaning "good" and "death."

39. On the tendency of the consequentialist to *redescribe* actions in terms of their intended results see Eric D'Arcy, *Human Acts: An Essay on their Moral Evaluation* (Oxford: Clarendon Press, 1963), pp. 1–40.

40. On God's innocence from evil see Jacques Maritain's superb study, *God and the Permission of Evil* (Milwaukee: Bruce, 1967).

41. On choosing in such a way that we preserve love for all human goods, not excluding some to the preference of others, see Germain Grisez and Russell Shaw, *Beyond the New Morality: The Responsibilities of Freedom* (Notre Dame: University of Notre Dame Press, 1974).

42. Grisez develops the incommensurability of human goods most remarkably in his *Abortion: The Myths, the Realities, and the Arguments* (New York: Corpus, 1970), chap. 6.

43. The indissoluble unity of body and soul in man is developed quite eloquently and effectively by Ramsey in *Patient as Person.*

44. Dyck shows the Stoic character of the ethics of euthanasia in his "An Alternative to Euthanasia."

45. See the superb development of the idea in Herbert McCabe, *What Is Ethics All About?* (Washington: Corpus, 1969), pp. 19–25.

46. Dyck, "An Alternative to an Ethics of Euthanasia," pp. 101–102.

47. Karl Barth, *Evangelical Theology: An Introduction* (New York: Holt, Rinehart and Winston, 1963), p. 11.

48. See Gerald Leach, *The Biocrats* (Baltimore: Penguin, 1972), the chapter on birth defects.

49. Karnofsky, cited in *Time,* Nov. 3, 1961, p. 60.

50. Cited by Ramsey, *op. cit.,* p. 145.

51. Cited by Ramsey, *op. cit.,* p. 151.

52. Ramsey (*op. cit.*) continues: "The difference between only caring for the dying and acts of euthanasia is not a choice between in-

directly and directly willing and doing something. It is rather the important choice between doing something and doing nothing, or (better said) ceasing to do something that was begun in order to do something that is better because more fitting. In omission no human agent causes the patient's death, directly or indirectly. He dies his own death from causes that it is no longer merciful or reasonable to fight by means of possible medical interventions. Indeed, it is not quite right to say that we only care for the dying by an omission, by 'doing nothing' directly or indirectly. Instead, we cease doing what was once called for and begin to do precisely what is called for now. We attend and company with him in this, his very own dying, rendering it as comfortable and as dignified as possible" (p. 151).

53. On this distinction see Gerald Kelly S.J., "The Duty of Using Artificial Means of Preserving Life," *Theological Studies,* 11 (1950): 203–220, and "The Duty to Preserve Life," *Theological Studies,* 12 (1951): 550–556. Kelly provides a good survey of pertinent texts from the Church's magisterium.

54. Pius XII, "Address to the International Congress of Anesthesiologists," Nov. 24, 1957, in *Acta Apostolicae Sedis,* 49 (1957): 1033ff., and *The Pope Speaks,* 4 (1958): 398ff.

55. See Maguire, "The Freedom to Die," p. 192.

56. Richard McCormick, "To Save or Let Die," *America,* 130 (1974): 6–10, at 8. This essay was also printed in *Journal of the American Medical Association,* 229 (1974): 172–176, and summarized in McCormick's "Notes on Moral Theology," *Theological Studies,* 36 (March 1975): 121–123.

57. *Ibid.*

58. *Ibid.*

59. See my "Ethics and Human Identity: The Challenge of the New Biology," p. 35.

60. McCormick, "To Save or Let Die," pp. 9–10.

61. See n. 29 above.

62. See Maguire, *Death by Choice,* p. 73, n. 42, with reference to McCormick's "Notes on Moral Theology," *Theological Studies* 34 (March, 1973): pp. 70–74.

63. See Dyck, "An Alternative to an Ethics of Euthanasia," pp. 111–112. The articulation here differs somewhat from his.

64. Thomas C. Oden, "Beyond an Ethic of Immediate Sympathy," *Hastings Center Report,* 6 (February 1976): 14.

65. See Roy Branson and Kenneth Casebeer, "Obscuring the Role of the Physician," *Hastings Center Report,* 6 (February 1976): 8–10.

66. He ruled the "ordinary-extraordinary" discussion not viable as legal distinctions.

67. E.g., Richard McCormick, as quoted by *Washington Post,* Apr. 3, 1976.

68. From the text of the court's ruling as given in Morriss County (N.J.) *Daily Record,* Apr. 1, 1976.

69. See Dr. McCarthy DeMere's comments in *Washington Post,* Apr. 3, 1976.

70. Oden, *art. cit.,* p. 14.

7: Death, Dying, and Organ Donation

Among the provisions of the Uniform Anatomical Gift Act is the following:

> The time of death shall be determined by a physician who attends the donor at his death, or, if none, the physician who certifies the death. This physician shall *not* participate in the procedures for removing or transplanting a part.[1]

The significance of this provision is that it establishes a legal procedure for protecting the dignity of the dying person.

In our legitimate desire to provide a suitable organ for one human being, whose life can be enhanced, perhaps saved, and whose health can in some measure be restored by transplant surgery, we must strenuously resist any temptation to diminish our care of a dying person because he is a prospective donor. It is for this reason that the World Medical Assembly, at a 1968 meeting in Sydney, Australia, accepted, as a matter of principle, complete separation of authority and responsibility between the physician or group of physicians who are responsible for the care of the dying person who is a prospective donor and the physician or group of physicians who are responsible for the care of the person in need of an organ transplant. This practice is commonly accepted, as it ought to be, by the medical community.

In the practical order, our rightful concern to ensure the dignity of the dying person is paralleled, or *ought* to be paralleled, by a concern in the intellectual order when we reflect on the meaning of death and on the criteria that are used to determine when a person is dead. Paul Ramsey has forcefully made this point, and it is imperative that we pay heed to what he said.

> If in the practical order we need to separate between the physician who is responsible for the care of a prospective donor, and the physician who is responsible for a prospective recipient, do we not need in the intellectual order to keep the question of the definition of death equally discrete from the use of organs in transplantations? If only the physician responsible for a dying man should make the determination that he has died, with no "help" from the medical team that has in its care a man who needs a borrowed organ, should not also the definition of death and the tests for it that he uses be ones that he thinks are sound or were agreed to by the profession without having transplantation in view? There would be too little protection of life attained in the practical order by entirely separating the authority and responsibility of the teams of physicians if the definition of death and the tests for it have already been significantly invaded by the requirements of transplant therapy. If no person's death should *for this purpose* be hastened, then the definition of death should not *for this purpose* be updated, or the procedures for stating that a man has died be revised as a means of affording easier access to organs.[2]

In calling attention to this passage I want to stress how necessary it is for us to heed the point it makes, and that point is our obligation to respect and care for our fellow human beings, especially those who are dying. Today, because of developments in the medical sciences and associated technologies, it is becoming more and more difficult to die and more and more difficult to determine when we have in our midst a living human being or a lifeless corpse. Contemporary concern to redefine "death" and establish criteria for determining when a human being is no longer alive has been caused, in large measure, by this twofold difficulty. But it would be foolish to hide from the fact that endeavors to "update death" have not also been influenced by the enormous strides in transplant surgery. Today, many people can be helped to live healthy lives *if* they can be provided with "new" vital organs, and a major source for such organs is the bodies of the recently deceased[3] and those who will soon become deceased.

Thus the need to secure organs for transplant surgery has affected the efforts to determine more adequately the criteria for telling when a person has died—so much, indeed, that the purpose of a major symposium was to define more clearly "the 'moment of death' *so that* those sick people who need transplanted tissues will not be sacrificed because of a lack of a clear definition as to when the donor has died."[4] Indeed, there has been, at times, a notable failure to distinguish properly between the living and the dead in the need to secure organs.

Carl E. Wassmuth and Bruce M. Steward have written that "when death occurs *or in the alternative when death has been declared inevitable,* the circulation and the respiration may be maintained by artificial means" to give surgeons time to remove the required organs.[5] And even Beecher, whose pioneering work on the ethics of human experimentation merits the attention and gratitude of everyone who is anxious to safeguard the dignity and transcendent moral worth of human beings, has declared: "Can society afford to discard the tissues and organs of hopelessly unconscious patients when they could be used to restore the otherwise hopelessly ill, but still salvageable individual?"[6]

The temptation to introduce transplant surgery and the need for vital organs into a discussion of the criteria for determining when a human being is no longer alive must be vigorously resisted. Even more strenuously ought we to reject efforts to blur the distinction between the living and dead and to reckon among the dead those dying but still living persons who are "hopelessly unconscious" and incapable of sapient and cognitive functions.[7] We must constantly remind ourselves, as Ramsey does, that "a patient whose death is 'imminent' or who is irreversibly dying is not yet dead."[8] We must recognize, as G. B. Giertz puts it, that "a person dying is still a person living."[9]

Care for the dying and respect for their humanity are cardinal principles that must govern our actions with respect to transplant surgery with vital organs that are to be donated by a deceased person and/or his family. Thus in thinking about death and in revising the criteria that determine when a person is dead the principal effort ought to be to make sure that "persons who have not died shall continue to be cared for and that persons who have died need not have 'life' sustaining measures inflicted upon their unburied corpses, needlessly and at great expense to their families."[10] The transplantation of vital organs must remain, in relation to our care for the dying and our efforts to determine when this care is no longer called for because the dying have died, "a secondary problem which must not interfere with the search for a more accurate definition of death," a point emphasized by Jean Hamburger.[11]

Determining When a Person Has Died

In "The Prolongation of Life," Pope Pius XII stressed that determination of death is a scientific question: "It is in the physician's domain . . . to give a clear and precise definition of death and of the 'moment of death' of a patient who dies without regaining consciousness."[12] Not long ago, before the sophisticated technologies that can now maintain vital functions artificially in the hope that eventually the patient will be able to carry them out spontaneously (even if assisted by implanted pacemakers, transplanted organs, or in an artificial respirator), it was not difficult for the scientific community, represented by the attending physician, to tell when a person was dead. He no longer breathed, his heart no longer pumped blood through his body, he no longer responded to stimuli. Today, however, this is not always the case. Persons who are "clinically dead," that is, persons who are no longer breathing and whose heart has stopped, can be revived or resuscitated; persons who are in a coma and unable to nourish themselves can be fed through tubes, so that they will not lose the ability to breathe and to circulate blood. But when are efforts to revive the clinically dead and to nourish the comatose reasonable medical interventions that must be taken if we are properly to discharge our obligation to protect the goods of life and health in our neighbor? The effort to answer this question has in large measure been responsible for the recent attempts to "update death."

Paul Ramsey has distinguished three schools of thought with respect to the criteria that should be used for determining when death has occurred.[13] The first, which has not been accepted by any responsible community of scientists, though it has received considerable popular attention, holds that human death means brain death and that the test for determining it is exclusively (or almost exclusively) a flat electroencephalograph. The second, which is represented by the famous *ad hoc* committee of Harvard Medical School and is reflected in a 1968 declaration of the World Medical Association, takes the meaning of death, philosophically, to be brain death, but it insists that several types of medical tests, in addition to the electroencephalograph, be employed to determine whether brain death has occurred. For instance, the World Medical Association's declaration maintains:

> The point of death of the different cells and organs is not so important as the certainty that the process has become irreversible by whatever techniques of resuscitation . . . may be employed. This determination will be based on clinical judgment supplemented if necessary by a number of diagnostic aids of which the electroencephalograph is currently the most helpful. However, no single technological criterion is entirely satisfactory in the present state of medicine nor can any one technological procedure be substituted for the overall judgment of the physician.[14]

The third school of thought differs from the other two in defining death not by brain death but as "the cessation of *integrated* life functions."[15] In this view, death is not simply the cessation of brain activity, as it is not simply the cessation of respiration or the circulation of blood. This is a traditional view of death, according to which it is not the notion of death that needs updating but rather the criteria for determining when death has occurred.

As noted, the first school of thought is not advocated by any responsible group. Ramsey believes, and for good reason, that the differences between the second and third groups are more theoretical than practical. "There is not so much difference between them," he writes,

> if we remember that doctors are not theoreticians debating the meaning of death but practical men primarily concerned to establish agreed-upon procedures for stating that death has occurred. Various sets of criteria are currently being proposed by committees of physicians. The

> discussion focuses on the procedures for determining that
> a man has died. . . . While among . . . physicians as well
> as the public at large there is a good deal of talk about
> brain death, it is safe to say that for the medical profes-
> sion death operationally means what is stated by the use
> of sound and sufficient criteria for telling when a man
> has died. These are almost always manifold tests or pro-
> cedures, not solely brain tests, if by the latter EEG is
> meant. . . . We should therefore take the current dis-
> cussions of death to be practical proposals for revising
> the procedures for stating that death has occurred, and
> not as discussions of the theoretical meaning of death.
> So understand, I am emboldened to suggest that the vari-
> ous accounts of how death might better be reckoned are
> not proposing anything very startling.[16]

I believe the notion that death consists in the cessation of integrated life functions is still the best notion and that the relevance of the tests advocated by such bodies as the World Medical
Association and the Harvard Medical School *ad hoc* committee is
best understood with reference to this definition. An immediate
effect of brain death is the inability to breathe spontaneously,
and this in turn results in the stopping of the heart. Since a
respirator can mechanically fill the lungs with oxygen and thereby
enable the heart to keep pumping, these "vital" operations can
at times be carried out in the body of a corpse. The purpose of
the diagnostic criteria for determining brain death is to help attending physicians realize that the continued use of a respirator
is no longer obligatory, since the person has died and therefore
no longer has the capacity for integrated functioning of heart,
lungs, and brain. This is the sole purpose, as many ethicists see
it, of the criteria for determining when brain death has occurred.
No one ought ever be declared dead simply because of a flat
electroencephalograph; no one ought ever be declared dead so
long as he is able to respirate spontaneously. But a comatose person who has no possibility ever to regain the capacity for spontaneous respiration, which can be ascertained by employing the
various tests to determine brain death, has already died; the integrated functioning of brain, heart, and lungs is no longer possible.

What must above all be resisted is the tendency to declare a
person legally dead when there is a flat EEG or when the various
diagnostic procedures have shown that the cortex of the brain,

the site of "higher" mental functions, is no longer operative, although the midbrain and brainstem are still functioning. A person in this condition is in the process of dying and no efforts to "save" him need be taken; in fact, it is morally wrong to impose such noncurative and death-prolonging procedures on him and his family. A person who is in this condition is dying and ought to be allowed to die. But such a person is still a living human person, not a recently deceased person, and therefore is not to be regarded as a repository of organ tissues.

Consenting to Organ Donation from Cadavers

Another major consideration in the use of vital organs of the recently deceased in transplant surgery—unless we wish to move into a society in which the "harvesting" of such organs becomes routine, which I do not think we wish to do[17]—is an adequately informed and reasonably free consent.[18] Here we must pause to ask why such consent is needed. After all, whose "property" is the body of the deceased, with its organs? The answer to this question is difficult, but perhaps we can find a starting point and a source for thinking deeply and seriously about the questions raised by using vital parts of the recently deceased in organ transplantation in the teaching embodied in the ethical and legal tradition of Western civilization, which is rooted in the Judeo-Christian view of the meaning of human existence.

According to this tradition, the body of a deceased person, with its organs, is not to be considered "property" at all, or not as property in the usual sense in which that term is employed. The words of a Rhode Island court in a case tried in 1872 are instructive:

> There is a duty imposed by the universal feelings of mankind to be discharged by someone towards the dead; a duty, and we may also say a right, to protect from violation; and a duty on the part of others to abstain from violation. . . . Although the body is not property in the usually recognized sense of the word, we may yet consider it as a sort of *quasi* property, to which certain persons may have rights, as they have duties to perform towards it arising out of our common humanity. . . . The person having charge of it [the body of a deceased human being]

cannot be considered as owner of it in any sense whatsoever; he holds it only as a sacred trust for the benefit of
all who from family or friendship have an interest in
its period.[19]

The legal doctrine that the body of a deceased person is the quasi property of that person's family and friends is, in essence, an affirmation that this body is *not* property to be disposed of, to be bartered or sold to the highest bidder. As Ramsey has noted, "The door to property in bodies in a commercial sense was paradoxically barred and bolted by the doctrine [that the body of a deceased human being is] quasi property!"[20]

Something deeply significant for our lives as human beings, as animals whose animality differs radically from that of other animals,[21] is at stake here. The value in question is the very same value that is imperiled by cannibalism—and the value behind civilized man's abhorrence of cannibalism. It is the value of our existence as persons whose personal being, whose dignity—indeed sanctity—is inescapably a *bodied* being, a *bodied* dignity, a *bodied* sanctity. The body of a human being, a human person, is not an instrument or tool; it is not subpersonal or subhuman, as the advocates of "creative intervention" in control of birth and death would have it.[22] To be a human being is not to be a spirit dwelling in a material body, somewhat as an actor "dwells" in ths costumes and makeup of the character he portrays. We are *not* incarnate spirits but living animals of a special kind. My body, your body, is not a costume that I or you put on; it is not an instrument that we use. My body is in truth "me," as your body is indeed "you."

Arrogantly to slight someone or viciously to strike him in the face is not to exert force on some material entity, accidentally and temporally linked to that someone; it is to do violence to a human person. We—you and I and every human being who has ever lived—*are* our bodies, and our bodies are not "property" that we possess or that anyone else possesses. That is the root reason why we cannot rightfully mutilate our bodies and why it would be wrong for me, here and now, to pluck out my eyes or cut off my nose or chop off my arm.[23]

The body of a deceased person, a corpse or cadaver, is not, of course, a body-person; it is an assemblage of disparate parts no longer unified in a living being. As Thomas Aquinas observed, a corpse or cadaver is not even a body; it is termed such only by equivocation.[24] Yet the corpse of a human being has real symbolic value. It reminds us that there was once in our midst a fellow man. It reminds us that our existence as humans is a co-existence and that to be human is to be *with* other humans. It symbolizes our common humanity and reminds us that what makes us beings of moral and transcendent worth is not uniquely mine or yours, not some private and individual possession, but something we share in common, in which we all participate, namely, our being as humans. It is for this reason that the bodies of the deceased are not to be the feast of birds or objects for commerce. The corpse of a deceased human being indeed has symbolic value, and man is unique as the symbol-using and symbol-making animal.

This is why consent must be secured for utilizing the organs of the deceased person in transplant surgery. This consent ought first to be sought from the dying person himself, and the Uniform Anatomical Gift Act, in seeking to reform a legal system that gives primary rights to the body of the deceased to the next of kin, is reaffirming the value affirmed in that legal system, namely, the deceased's body is not to be considered a commercial object, an item for barter. In giving priority to the explicit wishes of a person on the disposition of his own corpse and vital organs over the desires of his next of kin, that Act continues the ethical and legal tradition behind the common-law system it seeks to correct, for it tells us that we have a duty to let persons be themselves, that we are not to violate our fellow men, that we are not to regard their cadavers as commercial commodities or objects, that we are not to compete for their bodies as dogs do over bones.

Ideally, of course, consent to use the vital organs of a recently deceased person is best secured if that person has given such consent during his life, and preferably before he has been brought into an emergency room, the victim of an untimely and ghastly accident. In most instances, however, consent is not thus obtained or obtainable. Most often it is necessary to secure consent from relatives or friends, when they themselves are in a state of great anxiety or grief or shock. This calls for one of the greatest human endeavors: suffering and being compassionate with these relatives and friends, sharing their sorrow as they wait helplessly for word that one they love is no longer capable of sharing with them his life and love and hopes, and even his pain, and refraining from making their agony more cruel by making a nuisance of oneself. Yet it is a task that can be carried out well. It deepens our understanding of ourselves and the preciousness of the life we share, which is ebbing from the one whose organs can enable one of his brothers or sisters to preserve that life and, with it, the memory of this person, who, with his family and friends, has helped make it possible.

Conclusion

Since it is now possible for many persons to be helped by organ grafts, everyone should give very serious thought to "willing" his organs to them after death. We can sign a donor card, in conformity with the Uniform Anatomical Gift Act, making a gift of our eyes or kidneys or liver or heart to enable other persons, suffering from various ailments, to preserve the good of life and overcome their disabilities.

I believe that a gift of this kind expresses the covenant of love that God wills to share with us and wills us to share with others. Through a gift of this kind we can respond to his call to choose life, and, like him, we can live both with and for our fellow words.

Chapter 7

1. "Uniform Anatomical Gift Act, Section 7 (b)," as printed in Alfred M. Sadler, Jr., M.D., Blair L. Saddler, LL. B., and E. Blythe Stason, J.D., "The Uniform Anatomical Gift Act: A Model for Reform," *Journal of the American Medical Association,* 206 (Dec. 9, 1968): 2501–2506, at 2506.

2. Paul Ramsey, *The Patient as Person* (New Haven: Yale University Press, 1970), p. 103.

3. Henry K. Beecher, "Scarce Resources and Medical Advancement," *Daedalus* (Spring 1969), special issue on "Ethical Aspects of Human Experimentation," pp. 295–296.

4. Ramsey refers to this symposium in *op. cit.,* p. 104.

5. Carl E. Wassmuth and Bruce M. Steward, "Medical and Legal Aspects of Human Organ Transplantation," *Cleveland-Marshall Law Review*, 14 (1963): 466–467.

6. Beecher, *art. cit.*, p. 294. See the reply to Beecher (in the same issue of *Daedalus*) by Hans Jonas, "Philosophical Reflections on Human Experimentation," 220–245. See also Ramsey, *op. cit.*, pp. 106–109.

7. See the discussion in chap. 6.

8. Ramsey, *op. cit.*, p. 75.

9. G. B. Giertz, in G. E. W. Wolstenholme and Maeve O'Connor, eds., *Ethics in Medical Progress: With Special Reference to Transplantation* (Ciba Foundation Symposium) (Boston: Little, Brown, 1966), p. 147.

10. Ramsey, *op. cit.*, p. 105.

11. Jean Hamburger, in Wolstenholme and O'Connor, *op. cit.*, p. 206.

12. *Acta Apostolicae Sedis*, 45 (1957): 1027–1033.

13. Ramsey, *op. cit.*, pp. 63–98.

14. Declaration of the World Medical Association meeting in Sydney, Australia, Aug. 7, 1968.

15. Ramsey, *op. cit.*, pp. 63–65. See also Vincent J. Collins, M.D., "Limits of Medical Responsibility in the Prolongation of Life: A Guide to Decision—A Dying Score," *Journal of the American Medical Association*, 206 (1968): 390.

16. Ramsey, *op. cit.*, p. 66.

17. See Ramsey, *op. cit.*, pp. 198–215. Ramsey does not see anything inherently wrong in the routine salvaging of cadavers for vital organs. I think that he is right. Still, I believe that the symbolic transformation that such a policy would effect would inevitably lead to a lessening of respect for the value of human persons and that therefore this policy ought not be put into effect. In other words, teological or consequentialistic considerations are pertinent here.

18. On this subject see Ramsey, *op. cit.*, chap. 1, and chap. 1 above.

19. Pierce v. Swan Point Cemetery, 10 R.I. 227, 237, 238 (1872).

20. Ramsey, *op. cit.*, p. 205.

21. See Mortimer Adler, *The Difference of Man and the Difference It Makes* (New York: Meridian, 1968).

22. A pejorative attitude toward the human body and biological life

is manifest in the writings of those who extol human creativity and the right of moral man to intervene "creatively" into his biology to achieve birth and death by choice. See Fletcher's *Morals and Medicine* (Boston: Beacon Press, 1956) and Daniel Maguire's "The Freedom to Die" in *New Theology No. 10,* ed. Martin Marty and Dean Peerman (New York: Macmillan, 1973).

23. It is, of course, morally legitimate to permit one's members to be mutilated or dismembered if their mutilation or dismemberment is an inescapable element of an act of healing the whole body-person. In such acts the evil of mutilation is not properly intended by the agent nor is it the thrust of the action.

24. Thomas Aquinas, *Summa Theologiae,* I, 78, 2, ad 3.

Index